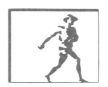

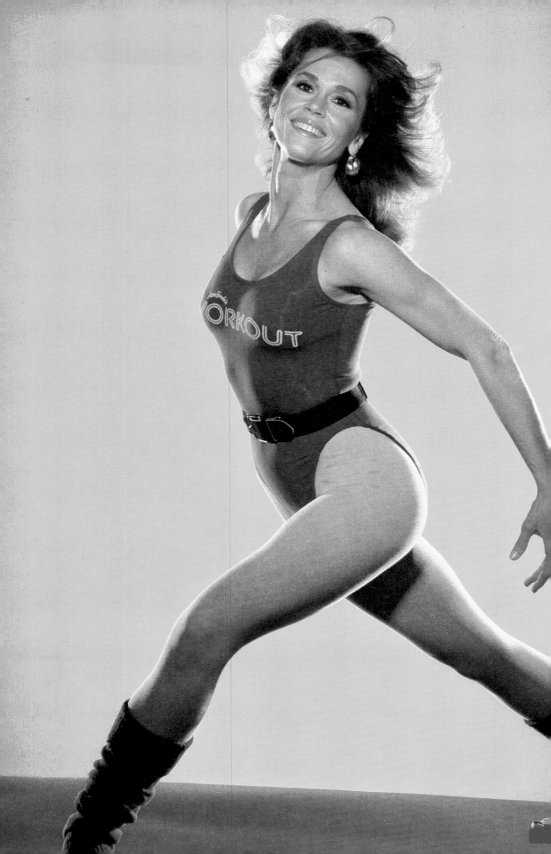

JANE FONDA'S
Year of
Fitness & Health
1984

Photographs by Dick Zimmerman
Drawings by Loren Clapp

SIMON AND SCHUSTER • NEW YORK

10   9   8   7   6   5   4   3   2   1

ISBN 0-671-46998-3

ACKNOWLEDGMENTS

The author gratefully acknowledges permission to adapt and reprint the recipes on these pages from the following cookbooks:

The Ashram Recipe Collection, The Ashram: pages 27 (top), 41 (bottom), 55 (bottom), 81 (all), 97 (both), 125 (both), 153 (bottom). The Ashram is a small health retreat in California that I have enjoyed. A copy of their recipe collection can be obtained by writing to The Ashram, P.O. Box 8, Calabasas, California 91302.

The Best Chance Diet by Joe D. Goldstrich, M.D., F.A.C.C.; © 1982 Humanics Limited, Atlanta, Georgia: page 109 (bottom).

Laurel's Kitchen—A Handbook for Vegetarian Cookery and Nutrition by Laurel Robertson, Carol Flinders, and Bronwen Godfrey; copyright 1976 Nilgiri Press, Petaluma, California: pages 39, 53, 109 (top), 111, 137, 165 (top), 167, 181 (bottom).

Let's Cook It Right by Adelle Davis; copyright 1947 © 1962 by Harcourt, Brace, Jovanovich, Inc., renewed 1975 by Frank Vernon Sieglinger. Reprinted by permission of the publisher: page 69.

The Natural Foods Cookbook by Beatrice Trum Hunter; copyright © 1961 by Beatrice Trum Hunter, reprinted by permission of Simon & Schuster, Inc.: pages 55 (top), 67 (bottom), 95 (middle and bottom), 139, 165 (bottom).

The Natural Foods Epicure by Nancy Albright; © 1983 by Nancy Albright, reprinted by permission of Rodale Press, Inc., Emmaus, Pennsylvania 18049: pages 27 (bottom), 41 (top), 83 (both), 181 (top).

CONTENTS

NEW BEGINNINGS

This is the start of a new year, 1984. I suggest that this year you *stop* hopping from one new diet to another, that you *stop* wishing you looked this way and felt that way, that you *stop* feeling guilty if you binge once in a while.

I suggest, instead, that you accept the health challenges offered each month of this new year and that you make a serious commitment to increase the *amount* of exercising you do.

If you do this, I promise you will feel better and look better by the end of 1984.

Our goal this year is quite basic: I want you to become more familiar with different types of exercise and I want you to shift to a low-fat, low-salt, low-sugar, low—animal-protein, high—complex-carbohydrate diet. You'll find out why as the year progresses.

In advocating this approach to eating, I am joining with the doctors, scientists and health experts who all agree that this is the healthiest way to eat and the best therapy for weight loss, diabetes, heart disease, cancer, arthritis and just plain wrinkles and bloat.

Let me explain specifically what I have done in this calendar:

EXERCISES: Each month I will focus on a different body part, giving exercises that strengthen and tone those muscles and other exercises that increase their flexibility. For January, concentrate on aerobics and stretching. You should continue these exercises throughout the year in addition to working on the specific muscle groups that will follow. Remember that there is no such thing as "spot reducing." If you want to lose fat you must do aerobic types of activities that burn the fat stores from all over your body. But in addition to burning up fat you should be building up and toning muscle tissue. Muscles are an important factor in weight loss. Muscle tissue is an *active* tissue which metabolizes almost 90 percent of the calories we consume. In addition, muscle tissue continues to burn calories even after you've stopped exercising.

Fat, on the other hand, is an *inactive* tissue. It burns few calories. In other words, the more fat you burn up through aerobic exercise and the more muscles you develop through repeated movements of isolated muscle groups, the more you will metabolize (burn up) the calories you consume.

Most diets are actually counter-productive. They slow down your metabolism and reduce muscle tissue. When you go off the diet (I've never known anyone who could stick to one) it's mainly fat you're putting on, not muscle, so you're worse off than when you started.

A great bonus of exercise is that it reduces your appetite: When your blood-sugar level drops, you feel hungry. If you exercise regularly, your blood-sugar level remains stable and there will be less insulin in your blood because your muscles use proportionately more fat than sugar as fuel. Insulin is what causes the blood-sugar level to drop precipitously, thereby making you feel hungry.

As I emphasize in my Workout Book, a proper exercise program must include:

- Aerobics—for cardiovascular fitness and to burn calories
- Repetition—to promote muscle tone and strength, and to burn calories
- Stretching—for increased flexibility

You should exercise at least three times a week, but you will lose weight much faster by doing your exercises four or five times a week. Forty-five to sixty minutes a day is ideal but twenty minutes is better than nothing.

If you have not been able to resist your favorite dessert or extra piece of bread, *don't feel guilty.* Everybody needs to binge now and again and being guilty about it will only make you more anxious and more apt to continue on a binge. Instead, and *I can't stress this enough,* just work out more strenuously the next day and you'll burn off the extra calories.

Never go for rapid weight loss. Your body will rebel sooner or later and you'll just put the pounds back on—faster. Instead, cut down a little on the amount you eat (say, 500 calories a day)—especially salt, fat and sugar—and increase your exercising. With this method your weight loss will be slow, but sure and steady. You will be losing fat, increasing muscle and developing a metabolism that, in time, will allow you to eat more without gaining weight.

For the most part, I have not specified the exact length of time or number of repetitions for each exercise and stretch. It is up to you to gauge your limits. Start easy and increase both your total time and number of repetitions each week. Keep track of the time spent exercising and the number of repetitions you are doing. Jot the figures down on your calendar each day. That way you can chart your progress. Try to work up a sweat, feel your muscles working to their maximum and your pulse accelerating.

It is important that you establish a steady, rhythmic tempo while doing the exercises and that you rest as little as possible between them. Also remember not to strain yourself. If at any time you feel excessive pain, stop and find out what is wrong before continuing.

HEALTH CHALLENGES: Each month I will ask you to accept a new health challenge. It may not be possible to be 100 percent perfect, but I hope you'll make a real effort to try to adjust your eating habits to these new approaches. If you *can* do them 100 percent, all the better! By the beginning of 1985, you'll wonder where you've been all your life.

I've included some favorite recipes that I've gathered along the road to good health. A glance at the Acknowledgments will give you a brief list of the best cookbooks I've found for healthful eating.

BASIC EATING ADVICE:
1. Eat only when you are really hungry.
2. Enjoy your food when you eat it.
3. Don't eat absent-mindedly, or out of boredom.
4. Chew well so that the digestive enzymes can begin their work *before* the food reaches the stomach.

Warning:
If you have sustained a recent injury or have chronic problems with your muscles or joints, please get professional advice before you begin any exercise program.

1983

JANUARY
S	M	T	W	T	F	S
						1
2	3	4	5	6	7	8
9	10	11	12	13	14	15
16	17	18	19	20	21	22
23	24	25	26	27	28	29
30	31					

FEBRUARY
S	M	T	W	T	F	S
		1	2	3	4	5
6	7	8	9	10	11	12
13	14	15	16	17	18	19
20	21	22	23	24	25	26
27	28					

MARCH
S	M	T	W	T	F	S
		1	2	3	4	5
6	7	8	9	10	11	12
13	14	15	16	17	18	19
20	21	22	23	24	25	26
27	28	29	30	31		

APRIL
S	M	T	W	T	F	S
					1	2
3	4	5	6	7	8	9
10	11	12	13	14	15	16
17	18	19	20	21	22	23
24	25	26	27	28	29	30

MAY
S	M	T	W	T	F	S
1	2	3	4	5	6	7
8	9	10	11	12	13	14
15	16	17	18	19	20	21
22	23	24	25	26	27	28
29	30	31				

JUNE
S	M	T	W	T	F	S
			1	2	3	4
5	6	7	8	9	10	11
12	13	14	15	16	17	18
19	20	21	22	23	24	25
26	27	28	29	30		

JULY
S	M	T	W	T	F	S
					1	2
3	4	5	6	7	8	9
10	11	12	13	14	15	16
17	18	19	20	21	22	23
24	25	26	27	28	29	30
31						

AUGUST
S	M	T	W	T	F	S
	1	2	3	4	5	6
7	8	9	10	11	12	13
14	15	16	17	18	19	20
21	22	23	24	25	26	27
28	29	30	31			

SEPTEMBER
S	M	T	W	T	F	S
				1	2	3
4	5	6	7	8	9	10
11	12	13	14	15	16	17
18	19	20	21	22	23	24
25	26	27	28	29	30	

OCTOBER
S	M	T	W	T	F	S
						1
2	3	4	5	6	7	8
9	10	11	12	13	14	15
16	17	18	19	20	21	22
23	24	25	26	27	28	29
30	31					

NOVEMBER
S	M	T	W	T	F	S
		1	2	3	4	5
6	7	8	9	10	11	12
13	14	15	16	17	18	19
20	21	22	23	24	25	26
27	28	29	30			

DECEMBER
S	M	T	W	T	F	S
				1	2	3
4	5	6	7	8	9	10
11	12	13	14	15	16	17
18	19	20	21	22	23	24
25	26	27	28	29	30	31

1984

JANUARY
S	M	T	W	T	F	S
1	2	3	4	5	6	7
8	9	10	11	12	13	14
15	16	17	18	19	20	21
22	23	24	25	26	27	28
29	30	31				

MAY
S	M	T	W	T	F	S
		1	2	3	4	5
6	7	8	9	10	11	12
13	14	15	16	17	18	19
20	21	22	23	24	25	26
27	28	29	30	31		

SEPTEMBER
S	M	T	W	T	F	S
						1
2	3	4	5	6	7	8
9	10	11	12	13	14	15
16	17	18	19	20	21	22
23	24	25	26	27	28	29
30						

FEBRUARY
S	M	T	W	T	F	S
			1	2	3	4
5	6	7	8	9	10	11
12	13	14	15	16	17	18
19	20	21	22	23	24	25
26	27	28	29			

JUNE
S	M	T	W	T	F	S
					1	2
3	4	5	6	7	8	9
10	11	12	13	14	15	16
17	18	19	20	21	22	23
24	25	26	27	28	29	30

OCTOBER
S	M	T	W	T	F	S
	1	2	3	4	5	6
7	8	9	10	11	12	13
14	15	16	17	18	19	20
21	22	23	24	25	26	27
28	29	30	31			

MARCH
S	M	T	W	T	F	S
					1	2
4	5	6	7	8	9	10
11	12	13	14	15	16	17
18	19	20	21	22	23	24
25	26	27	28	29	30	31

JULY
S	M	T	W	T	F	S
1	2	3	4	5	6	7
8	9	10	11	12	13	14
15	16	17	18	19	20	21
22	23	24	25	26	27	28
29	30	31				

NOVEMBER
S	M	T	W	T	F	S
				1	2	3
4	5	6	7	8	9	10
11	12	13	14	15	16	17
18	19	20	21	22	23	24
25	26	27	28	29	30	

APRIL
S	M	T	W	T	F	S
1	2	3	4	5	6	7
8	9	10	11	12	13	14
15	16	17	18	19	20	21
22	23	24	25	26	27	28
29	30					

AUGUST
S	M	T	W	T	F	S
			1	2	3	4
5	6	7	8	9	10	11
12	13	14	15	16	17	18
19	20	21	22	23	24	25
26	27	28	29	30	31	

DECEMBER
S	M	T	W	T	F	S
						1
2	3	4	5	6	7	8
9	10	11	12	13	14	15
16	17	18	19	20	21	22
23	24	25	26	27	28	29
30	31					

JANUARY

S	M	T	W	T	F	S
1	2	3	4	5	6	7
8	9	10	11	12	13	14
15	16	17	18	19	20	21
22	23	24	25	26	27	28
29	30	31				

EXERCISE—
AEROBICS

Jogging
Jumping Jacks
Step-ups
Inner Thigh and Back Stretch
Hamstring and Lower Back Stretch
Lower Back, Groin and Hamstring Stretch

HEALTH CHALLENGE—
IMPROVE YOUR FLEXIBILITY

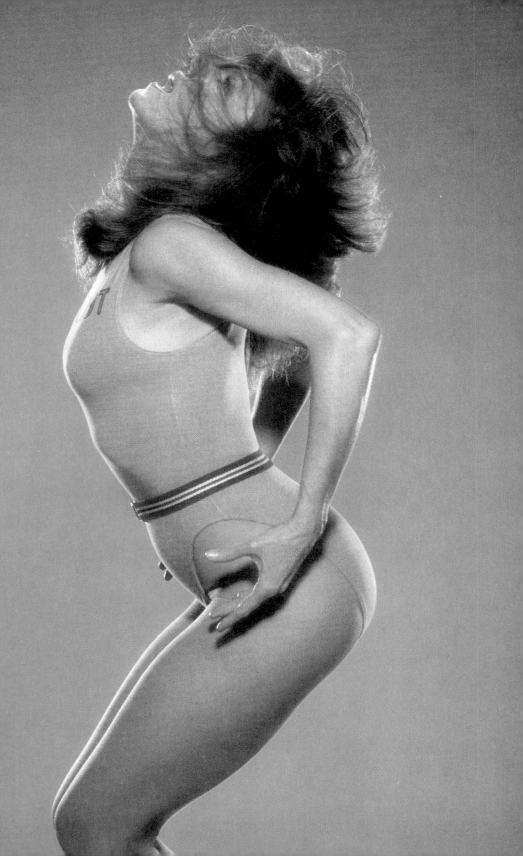

JANUARY

Exercise—AEROBICS

Start off this new year with a commitment to improving your cardiovascular fitness: the ability of your heart to pump more oxygen-carrying blood through your vascular system with fewer beats.

Aerobic exercise is the best way to do this. Walking briskly (up and down hills when possible), jogging, running, cross-country skiing, swimming, cycling, jumping rope and vigorous, non-stop exercise are aerobic activities. They are rhythmic, sustained and use the large muscle groups, particularly those in the hips and legs.

The rhythmic contractions of these large hip and leg muscles press against the blood vessels so that they send increased amounts of blood to the heart, making the heart muscle work harder.

Because aerobic exercise causes the heart to pump more blood it also increases the amount of oxygen available to our muscles (oxygen is carried through the body by the red blood cells). Without oxygen, our muscles cannot produce energy.

And remember: Aerobic exercise burns calories (approximately 100 calories every ten minutes), slims the hips, buttocks and thighs, and makes you feel vibrant and energetic.

Start with four minutes a day. Add one minute every week up to a maximum of thirty minutes a day, five times a week. That's a maximum. The minimum goal should be twelve to fifteen minutes three times a week.

Health Challenge—IMPROVE YOUR FLEXIBILITY

Flexibility is critical to overall fitness and can be achieved through stretching exercises. With patience, *anyone* can increase his or her flexibility.

Stretching increases our range of motion, keeps our muscles supple and improves circulation.

Many exercise enthusiasts, athletes and bodybuilders have great muscle tone and cardiovascular fitness but lack flexibility, making them more prone to injuries such as muscle strain, shinsplints and tendinitis.

Your stretch exercises should be done before and after any activity that causes tightness—jogging, bodybuilding or aerobic dance—to prepare your muscles for the work they are about to do and minimize the risk of hurting yourself.

Stretching should be done in a manner that is not stressful and is as relaxed as possible, in order to reduce muscular tension. Relaxed stretching done *regularly* will do more good than forcing yourself too far too fast. A muscle that is overstretched will tighten up.

Go into a stretch gradually and only as far as you can without strain. Hold it twenty to forty seconds. Breathe steadily the whole time. Release. Stretch again. Hold. Release. Try to increase the stretch very slightly each time. *And never hold your breath.* The shaded areas in the drawings of the stretch exercises indicate where you should be feeling the stretch.

JANUARY

	MORNING	AFTERNOON
1 SUNDAY	NEW YEAR'S DAY	
2 MONDAY		
3 TUESDAY		
4 WEDNESDAY		
5 THURSDAY		
6 FRIDAY		
7 SATURDAY		
8 SUNDAY		

Exercise—Aerobics
Health Challenge—Improve Your Flexibility

JOGGING

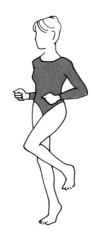

Jog in place. You should land on the balls of your feet and then work through the whole foot, making sure that your heels touch down on each step.

JUMPING JACKS

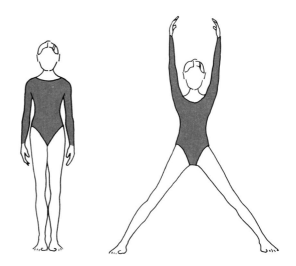

Stand with feet together, arms at your sides. Jump up and open your legs, as your arms swing out to the side and up over your head, landing with your legs as far apart as possible. Then jump up and land with your feet together as you bring your arms down to your sides again. Do this at a steady even pace.

JANUARY

	MORNING	AFTERNOON
9 MONDAY		
10 TUESDAY		
11 WEDNESDAY		
12 THURSDAY		
13 FRIDAY		
14 SATURDAY		
15 SUNDAY	MARTIN LUTHER KING'S BIRTHDAY	

Exercise—Aerobics
Health Challenge—Improve Your Flexibility

STEP-UPS

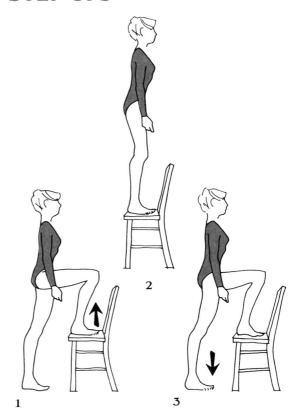

Get a good, sturdy chair or bench about fifteen to twenty inches high. Place your right foot flat on the chair. With your arms at your sides, step up so you are standing on the chair seat. Then step down to the floor with your right foot and bring your left foot down. On the next step-up, start with your left foot first and step down with your left foot first. Repeat for two minutes, working up to ten minutes. Maintain regular breathing. Increase the tempo as you can.

JANUARY

	MORNING	AFTERNOON
16 MONDAY		
17 TUESDAY		
18 WEDNESDAY		
19 THURSDAY		
20 FRIDAY		
21 SATURDAY		
22 SUNDAY		

Exercise—Aerobics
Health Challenge—Improve Your Flexibility

INNER THIGH AND BACK STRETCH

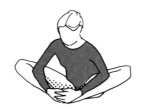 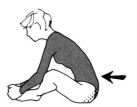

Sit on the floor and place the soles of your feet together. Hold on to your toes and, keeping your head up and back straight, press forward from your hips. To increase the stretch, gently place your elbows down against your lower legs. Hold. Breathe. Release slowly and repeat.

HAMSTRING AND LOWER BACK STRETCH

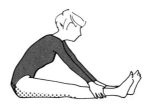 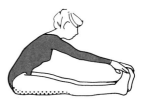

Sit with your legs together straight out in front of you, feet flexed. Bend forward from the hips as far as you can without strain, pressing the backs of the knees into the floor. Hold, breathing normally. Release for a moment, then repeat. Try to hold your toes during the stretch if you can.

JANUARY

	MORNING	AFTERNOON
23 MONDAY		
24 TUESDAY		
25 WEDNESDAY		
26 THURSDAY		
27 FRIDAY		
28 SATURDAY		
29 SUNDAY		

Exercise—Aerobics
Health Challenge—Improve Your Flexibility

LOWER BACK, GROIN AND HAMSTRING STRETCH

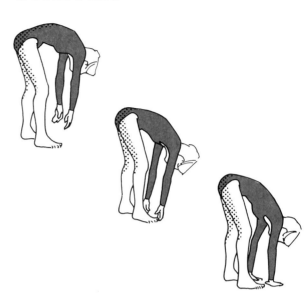

Stand with your feet a little more than hip-distance apart, toes pointed straight ahead. Slowly bend forward from the hips. Relax your neck and arms. Bend down until you feel a stretch up the back of your legs. These are the hamstring muscles and tendons. *Do not bounce,* but hold a steady stretch for twenty seconds. Bend your knees slightly to ease your lower back if necessary. You should feel relaxed. Then slowly roll back up and repeat.

JANUARY/FEBRUARY

	MORNING	AFTERNOON
30 MONDAY		
31 TUESDAY		
1 WEDNESDAY		
2 THURSDAY		
3 FRIDAY		
4 SATURDAY		
5 SUNDAY		

Exercise—Aerobics
Health Challenge—Improve Your Flexibility

Tofu Tomato Bakes ("Pizza")

If you like pizza as much as I do, here's a delicious low-calorie version.

Cut firm tofu into slices (3"x3"x¼").Drain well. (You may use defrosted frozen tofu for this recipe.) Brown lightly on both sides in a small amount of oil. Remove to a baking dish or cookie sheet. Top with tomato sauce, then sprinkle on minced garlic, sliced olives, mushrooms, green pepper, and grated cheese. Bake until cheese melts, or broil for a couple of minutes until vegetables are warm and cheese is melted.

Sprinkle with basil, oregano and thyme to taste.

Cashew Carrot Soup

2 *medium onions, sliced*
4 *tablespoons oil*
2 *cups coarsely shredded cabbage, turnip greens or Swiss chard*
2 *cups grated carrots*
1 *cup chopped apple*
5 *cups beef stock*
2 *tablespoons tomato paste*
⅓ *cup brown rice*
½ *cup coarsely chopped cashew nuts*
½ *cup raisins*
1 *to 1½ cups yogurt*
Salt, pepper to taste

Using a Dutch oven or heavy-bottomed pot, sauté onions in oil. Stir in greens and sauté a few minutes, then add the carrots and cook a minute or so longer. Stir in apples, beef stock and tomato paste. Bring mixture to a boil and add rice. Simmer, covered, for 35 to 40 minutes or until carrots are tender and rice is cooked.

Add cashew nuts and raisins and cook until raisins are "plumped." Season to taste. Serve each bowl of soup topped with a generous dollop of yogurt. Serves 4 to 6.

FEBRUARY

S	M	T	W	T	F	S
			1	2	3	4
5	6	7	8	9	10	11
12	13	14	15	16	17	18
19	20	21	22	23	24	25
26	27	28	29			

EXERCISE—
ARMS

Arm Circles
Deltoid Swing
Triceps Lifts
Praying Mantis
Triceps and Shoulder Stretch

HEALTH CHALLENGE—
AVOID SALT

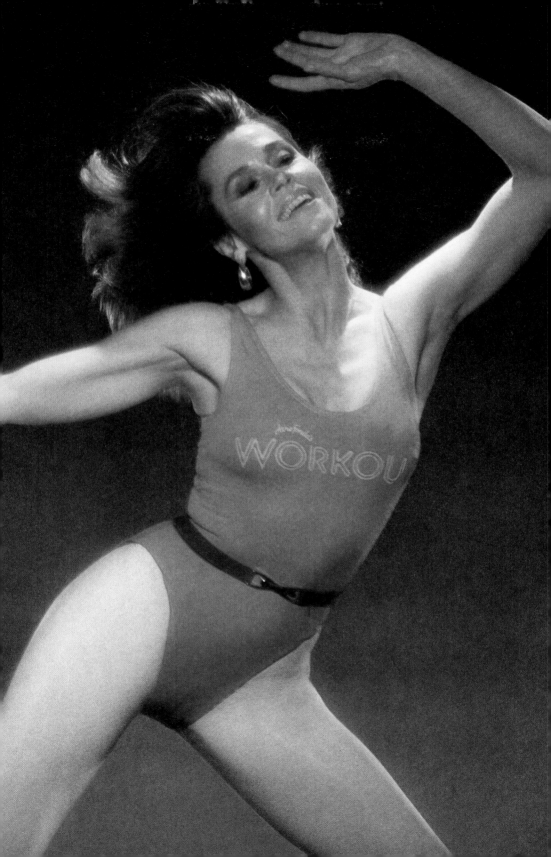

FEBRUARY

Exercise—ARMS

Arms can be beautiful when the muscles in the shoulders are rounded and defined. Women tend not to use their arms and upper bodies as strenuously as men; hence there is a tendency to lose muscular definition and develop "sagging" under the arms.

The shoulder muscle is the deltoid. The muscle that can tighten up the sagging underarm is the triceps.

Health Challenge—AVOID SALT

Sodium from salt and additives such as monosodium glutamate increases the risk of developing high blood pressure. Salt also causes fluid retention—which gives you that puffy look, stretches the skin, and adds weight.

There is enough salt in the foods you eat without your having to add more. Don't add it in cooking. Don't salt the food on your plate, and avoid processed foods, which tend to be highly salted. In time, as you cut back on salt, your taste buds will become much more alert to the subtle and delicious flavors in food.

Some recommended substitutes for salt:
- Vegit: A powdered herbal and vegetable salt substitute made by Gayelord Hauser available in health food stores.
- My father's recipe for homemade salt substitute:

HENRY FONDA'S SALT SUBSTITUTE

3 oz. powdered vegetable broth
¼ teaspoon garlic powder
⅛ teaspoon oregano
¼ teaspoon dill seed
¼ teaspoon paprika
¼ teaspoon honey fructose
¼ teaspoon margarine
½ teaspoon powdered kelp
⅛ teaspoon ground celery seed
¼ teaspoon Five-pepper blend
½ teaspoon dry mustard
Grated lemon peel to taste

Mix all ingredients and store in closed container in dry place.

- Kelp granules: This is a seaweed, an excel-
  lent source of calcium and other minerals.
  The powdered version doesn't taste as good
  so get the granules.
- Vegetable Broth Powders
- Miso: A soybean paste
- Tamari: Soy sauce

JANUARY/FEBRUARY

	MORNING	AFTERNOON
30 MONDAY		
31 TUESDAY		
1 WEDNESDAY		
2 THURSDAY		
3 FRIDAY		
4 SATURDAY		
5 SUNDAY		

Exercise—Arms
Health Challenge—Avoid Salt

ARM CIRCLES

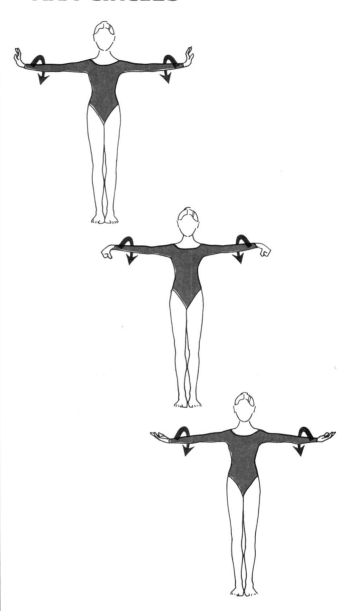

Stand with feet together, arms stretched out to the side just below shoulder level and slightly forward. Shoulders should be relaxed, stomach pulled in, buttocks squeezed tight. Circle both arms to the back 24 times with your hands flexed upward, 24 times with your knuckles flexed downward, 24 times with palms cupped upward.

FEBRUARY

	MORNING	AFTERNOON
6 MONDAY		
7 TUESDAY		
8 WEDNESDAY		
9 THURSDAY		
10 FRIDAY		
11 SATURDAY		
12 SUNDAY	LINCOLN'S BIRTHDAY	

Exercise—Arms
Health Challenge—Avoid Salt

DELTOID SWING

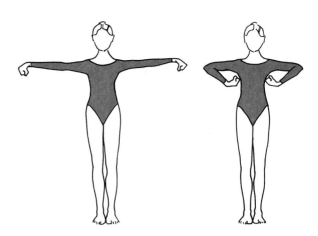

Stand with feet together, arms stretched out to the side, shoulder height, fists dropped down. In a steady, rhythmic tempo, bend your elbows bringing the fists in toward your body, breast height, and then out again. Keep your upper arms shoulder height the entire time.

TRICEPS LIFTS

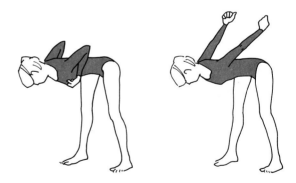

Stand with feet wide apart (you may bend your knees slightly). Bend forward, keeping your back flat, until your torso is parallel to the floor. Make fists with both hands close to your shoulders, elbows bent alongside your torso and pointing upward. Then straighten your arms and stretch them as high as possible behind you without letting them go out to the sides. Bring them in again and repeat this movement at a fairly rapid and rhythmic tempo until your muscles tire.

FEBRUARY

	MORNING	AFTERNOON
13 MONDAY		
14 TUESDAY	ST. VALENTINE'S DAY	
15 WEDNESDAY		
16 THURSDAY		
17 FRIDAY		
18 SATURDAY		
19 SUNDAY		

Exercise—Arms
Health Challenge—Avoid Salt

PRAYING MANTIS

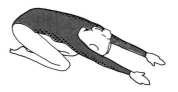

Sit back on your heels, knees hip-distance apart. Bend forward, placing your forehead and hands, palms down, on the floor. Slide or walk your forearms as far forward as you can while keeping your back and neck in a straight line. You should be looking toward your feet. You can increase the stretch by reaching forward alternately with one arm then the other, but keep your hips down on your heels and your forehead on the floor. Hold at the extreme position of the stretch then release.

TRICEPS AND SHOULDER STRETCH

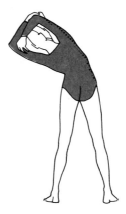

Stand with your feet a little more than hip-distance apart. Bring your arms up, crossing them behind your head and grasping each elbow with your hands. Gently pull your right elbow with the left hand as you bend slowly to the left side from your hips. You may bend your knees slightly. *Be sure your hips are forward and that your torso bends directly to the side without leaning forward—and don't arch your back.* Repeat to opposite side.

FEBRUARY

	MORNING	AFTERNOON
20 MONDAY	WASHINGTON'S BIRTHDAY OBSERVED	
21 TUESDAY		
22 WEDNESDAY	WASHINGTON'S BIRTHDAY	
23 THURSDAY		
24 FRIDAY		
25 SATURDAY		
26 SUNDAY		

Exercise—Arms
Health Challenge—Avoid Salt

Minestrone

1 onion, finely chopped
¼ cup olive oil
1½ cups chopped celery
4 cups grated fresh tomatoes (or 1 large can
  tomatoes with juice)
1 or 2 cups vegetable stock, if needed
½ cup chopped parsley
Dash pepper
1 or 2 bay leaves
1 teaspoon oregano
2 teaspoons basil
½ teaspoon rosemary
Dash garlic powder
2 cups or more, chopped and steamed nearly
  done: carrots, zucchini, broccoli, potatoes,
  green beans, green pepper, cabbage, peas,
  corn, sautéed mushrooms
1 cup cooked lima, kidney, pinto, black or
  garbanzo beans
½ cup raw whole wheat noodles or broken
  whole wheat spaghetti
½ cup cooked barley or whole wheat berries
Spinach and/or chard cut into bite-size pieces
Parmesan cheese (optional)

Sauté onion and celery in oil until soft. Add the tomatoes, parsley, seasonings and vegetable stock. Simmer the soup while you prepare whatever grains, beans and vegetables you wish to add. At least 30 minutes before serving, add the cooked beans, the raw noodles or spaghetti, and the cooked barley or wheat berries. Combine steamed vegetables with the soup about 10 minutes before serving. The greens should be added just 5 minutes before serving. Bring the soup to a boil, simmer a minute or two while correcting the seasonings. Garnish each bowl with a spoonful of Parmesan cheese. Makes about 10 cups.

FEBRUARY/MARCH

	MORNING	AFTERNOON
27 MONDAY		
28 TUESDAY		
29 WEDNESDAY	LEAP YEAR DAY	
1 THURSDAY		
2 FRIDAY		
3 SATURDAY		
4 SUNDAY		

Exercise—Arms
Health Challenge—Avoid Salt

Split Peas with Barley

This recipe can be cooked in a crockery pot.*

    2 tablespoons oil
    ¼ cup chopped onion
    ¼ cup chopped green pepper
    ¾ cup split peas
    ¼ cup soy grits
    ¾ cup pearl barley
3½ cups stock
    2 tablespoons chopped parsley
    3 tablespoons chopped fresh or 1 teaspoon
        dried dill
    1 teaspoon Vegit
Chopped fresh parsley

Heat oil in a heavy saucepan and sauté onion and green pepper for approximately 5 minutes. Add split peas, soy grits and barley, stirring constantly until they are coated with oil (approximately 3 minutes). Add stock, parsley, dill and Vegit.

Cover pot and simmer for approximately 1¼ hours or until barley is tender. Serve hot, garnished with chopped parsley. Serves 6.

* If using crockery pot, omit the preceding steps and proceed with method below.

Soak split peas for at least 4 hours in water to cover. Drain. Omit oil. Combine soaked split peas with remaining ingredients. Cook on low for 8 to 10 hours.

Parsley Dressing

Using 1 to 2 cups plain yogurt as a base, combine, to taste, a little safflower oil, hot mustard, Worcestershire sauce, honey, juice of ½ lemon, juice of 1 orange, freshly ground black pepper, and lots of finely chopped fresh parsley. Season with fresh dill weed and oregano. Use on any green salad. Yield: 1 to 2 cups.

MARCH

S	M	T	W	T	F	S
				1	2	3
4	5	6	7	8	9	10
11	12	13	14	15	16	17
18	19	20	21	22	23	24
25	26	27	28	29	30	31

EXERCISE—
PECTORALS

Shoulder and Chest Stretch
Push-ups
Front Arm Cross

HEALTH CHALLENGE—
DRINK MORE WATER

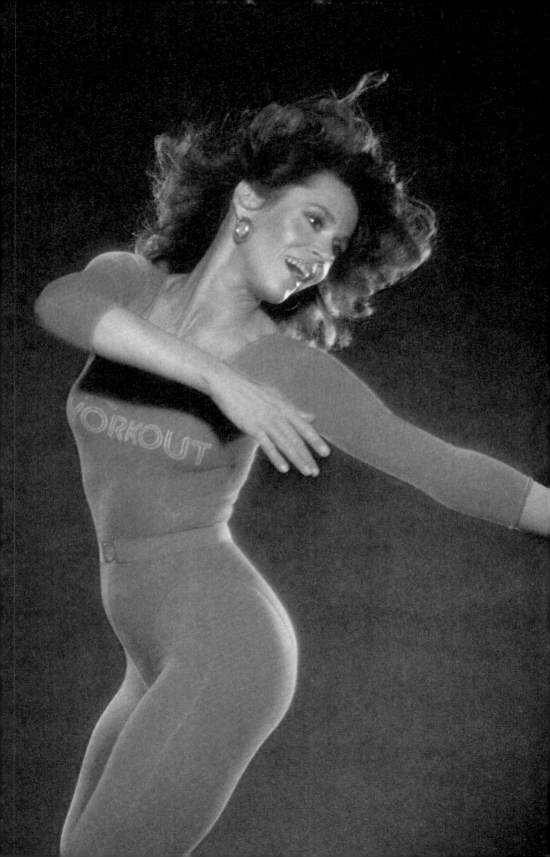

MARCH

Exercise—PECTORALS

Pectorals are the muscles in the upper chest that run from the shoulders to the breast. Building up the pectorals does not enlarge the breasts, but it does lift them and helps to create cleavage and lovely roundness over the chest bones.

Health Challenge—DRINK MORE WATER

Perhaps one of the most healthful things I will ask you to do this year is to drink more water, but you must continue to avoid salt, since salt will cause you to retain fluid. Water is the best natural diuretic there is. It will flush out your system, improve your skin and overall health.

Six to eight glasses daily is what you should aim for. Keep track of your drinks by noting them on your daily calendar. Some nutritionists believe it is best to drink water between meals instead of with them so that digestion will be most efficient.

I recommend drinking bottled water—natural or distilled—to avoid any possible pollutants that may exist in your area's water system.

If you travel a lot by plane and are bothered by jet lag, try my sure-fire remedy: Eat before leaving for the airport, not on the plane. Ask the stewardess to give you a pitcher of water with little or no ice and keep refilling it. Drink constantly (you may want an aisle seat!). When you arrive at your destination, have a light, healthy meal, do some stretches and if possible, take a short, brisk walk. People will wonder how you manage not to be tired.

FEBRUARY/MARCH

	MORNING	AFTERNOON
27 MONDAY		
28 TUESDAY		
29 WEDNESDAY		
1 THURSDAY		
2 FRIDAY		
3 SATURDAY		
4 SUNDAY		

Exercise—Pectorals
Health Challenge—Drink More Water

SHOULDER AND CHEST STRETCH

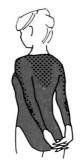

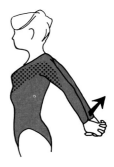

Stand with feet a few inches apart. Clasp your hands behind your back and, keeping your arms straight, lift them up behind you until you feel a stretch in the shoulders and chest. Hold, keeping your chest out, chin in and shoulders down.

MARCH

	MORNING	AFTERNOON
5 MONDAY		
6 TUESDAY		
7 WEDNESDAY	ASH WEDNESDAY	
8 THURSDAY		
9 FRIDAY		
10 SATURDAY		
11 SUNDAY		

Exercise—Pectorals
Health Challenge—Drink More Water

PUSH-UPS

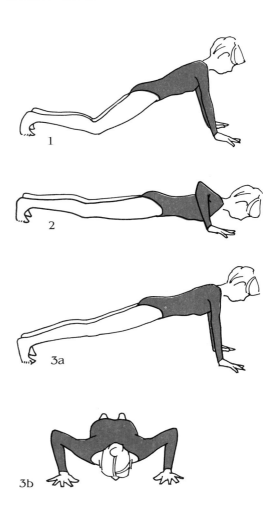

1. Start on your hands and knees with toes on the floor, hands parallel to each other a little more than shoulder-width apart. The wider apart your hands are, the more you work your pectoral muscles.

2. Keeping your knees on the floor, lower your body straight down as far as you can, then push yourself straight up to the starting position. Continue until your muscles tire. *Concentrate on keeping your back flat. Don't let your buttocks stick up.* Inhale as you lower, exhale as you push up.

3. As you develop strength in your arms and chest, try straight-leg push-ups.

Start slowly. Increase the number of push-ups gradually.

MARCH

	MORNING	AFTERNOON
12 **MONDAY**		
13 **TUESDAY**		
14 **WEDNESDAY**		
15 **THURSDAY**		
16 **FRIDAY**		
17 **SATURDAY**	ST. PATRICK'S DAY	
18 **SUNDAY**		

Exercise—Pectorals
Health Challenge—Drink More Water

FRONT ARM CROSS

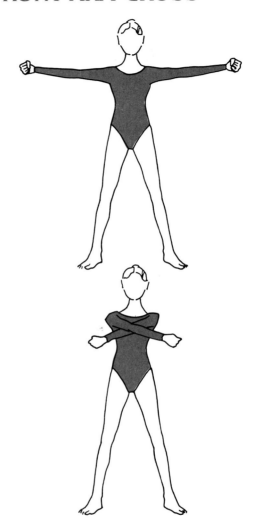

Stand up very straight with feet wide apart, stomach pulled in, buttocks tight and arms out to sides. Starting at waist height, criss-cross (cross, then open) your straight arms in front of your body with closed fists facing inward. Continue criss-crossing straight arms while raising them above your head, then lowering them slowly back down to waist level. Repeat 6 times. Then do 20 criss-crosses with arms at shoulder-height. The wider you open your arms before crossing them, the more you work your pectorals.

MARCH

	MORNING	AFTERNOON
19 MONDAY		
20 TUESDAY		
21 WEDNESDAY		
22 THURSDAY		
23 FRIDAY		
24 SATURDAY		
25 SUNDAY		

Exercise—Pectorals
Health Challenge—Drink More Water

Tofu Patties

½ onion, finely chopped
1 stalk celery, finely chopped
½ green pepper, finely chopped
2 tablespoons oil
1 package tofu (about 20 ounces)
1 egg, beaten
2 tablespoons whole wheat flour
2 tablespoons soy sauce
2 teaspoons curry powder or ½ cup grated
   Cheddar cheese
Wheat germ, or cornmeal, or sesame seeds

Sauté the onion, celery and green pepper in oil until soft. Drain the tofu in a strainer; then mash it with a fork and mix in the egg, flour, and soy sauce. Add vegetables and either the curry powder or the cheese. Form into small patties and roll them in the wheat germ. Brown on a griddle or skillet, or bake in a 350° oven. Makes about 2 dozen.

MARCH/APRIL

	MORNING	AFTERNOON
26 MONDAY		
27 TUESDAY		
28 WEDNESDAY		
29 THURSDAY		
30 FRIDAY		
31 SATURDAY		
1 SUNDAY		

Exercise—Pectorals
Health Challenge—Drink More Water

Pilau

4 tablespoons oil
1 onion, chopped
1 clove garlic, minced
1 cup brown rice, raw
2 cups seasoned stock, hot
3 tablespoons nutritional yeast (optional)
¼ teaspoon cloves, ground
3 cardamom seeds, crushed
½ teaspoon allspice, ground
½ teaspoon cinnamon, ground
¼ cup almonds, slivered
¼ cup raisins

Heat oil and sauté onion and garlic. Add rice and cook, stirring constantly until each grain is transparent. Dissolve yeast (if used) and spices in hot stock. Add ½ cup of stock to rice mixture. Cover and simmer gently, gradually adding rest of stock as liquid is absorbed. Add almonds and raisins. Rice should be tender in 30 to 40 minutes. Serves 6.

Tofu Hummus Plus

8 ounces tofu, drained, mashed with fork
½ cup tahini
1 tablespoon dark miso paste
3 tablespoons fresh-squeezed lemon juice
½ cup garbanzos, mashed (may use canned or fresh cooked)
2 teaspoons olive oil
1 teaspoon crushed basil leaves
1 tablespoon dry seasoning mix
½ teaspoon dulse flakes or powder
¼ teaspoon ground cumin
1 clove garlic, crushed (or ½ teaspoon garlic powder)

Combine all ingredients and mix well. Serve with crackers or chips.

APRIL

S	M	T	W	T	F	S
1	2	3	4	5	6	7
8	9	10	11	12	13	14
15	16	17	18	19	20	21
22	23	24	25	26	27	28
29	30					

EXERCISE—
WAIST

Side Pulls
Open Stride Floor Stretch
Standing Waist Stretch

HEALTH CHALLENGE—
CUT DOWN ON SUGAR

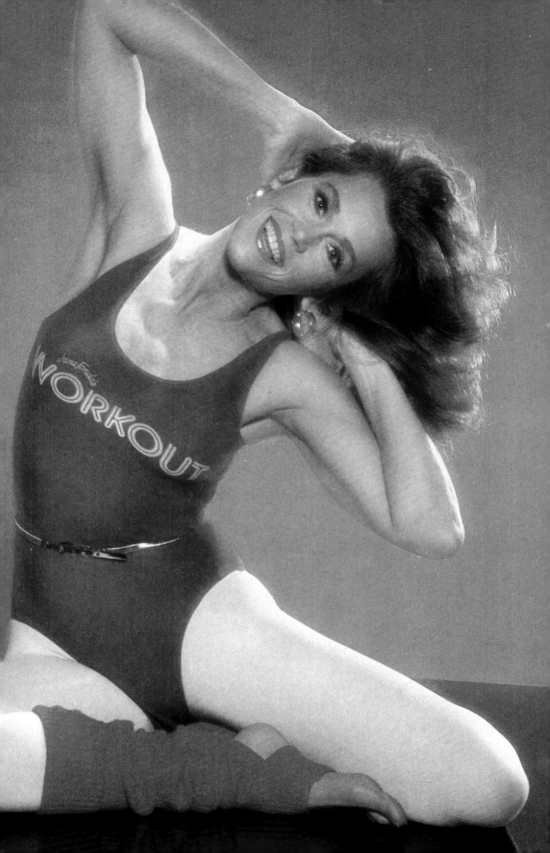

Exercise—WAIST

The Side Pulls I've chosen for this month are the best exercises for the waist I've ever found. They both stretch and tone the intercostal and oblique muscles of the waist. However, it is very easy to do them incorrectly. Here's what to look out for:

1. *Do not move your hips.* All the movement is in the upper body.
2. Legs are *wide* apart for balance.
3. Head and neck are relaxed.
4. Pull *straight to the side.* Be sure your shoulders are aligned with your hips, not twisting forward; that your hips are square to the front and tucked under. At the Workout, we ask students to imagine they're between two sheets of glass. If they lean forward or backward, the glass will break.

Health Challenge—CUT DOWN ON SUGAR

Take sugar off your grocery list, brown sugar too. Americans are now eating 130 pounds of sugar per person per year! This is more than a third of a pound daily for every woman, man and child. Besides being devoid of nutrients, sugar is a full-time promoter of tooth decay, obesity, heart disease and diabetes. Sugar is often listed on labels as corn syrup, dextrose, maltose, glucose and invert sugar. Stay away from it! This includes alcohol, which is extremely high in sugar. If you have problems such as high blood pressure, diabetes or heart disease, you shouldn't drink *any* alcohol. If you are healthy, limit yourself to a glass of wine or two beers a day.

If you need a sweetener, use uncooked honey, which besides containing copper, iron, calcium and potassium—in addition to other important minerals—and all nine essential amino acids, is a mild laxative and sedative as well. Pure maple syrup, apple juice, true fructose and date sugar are other healthful replacements for sugar.

There are times of day (usually the afternoon) when our blood-sugar level drops and we feel a need for a quick sugar-hit for energy. Protect yourself against the sugar urge by carrying an apple or other piece of fresh fruit. Raisins, sunflower seeds, raw almonds or carob drops will also do the trick. But stick with the fruit if you're trying to lose weight.

APRIL

	MORNING	AFTERNOON
1 SUNDAY	APRIL FOOL'S DAY	
2 MONDAY		
3 TUESDAY		
4 WEDNESDAY		
5 THURSDAY		
6 FRIDAY		
7 SATURDAY		
8 SUNDAY		

Exercise—Waist
Health Challenge—Cut Down on Sugar

SIDE PULLS

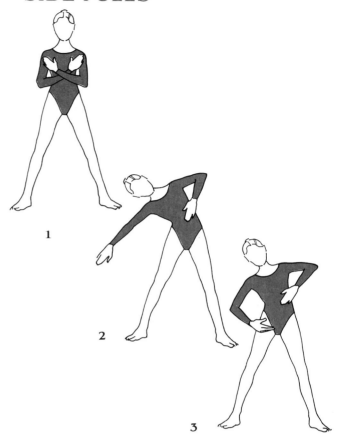

1. Stand with your feet a little more than hip-distance apart, stomach pulled in, buttocks tight, hands crossed in front of your torso, palms facing your body.

2. Pull over to the right, reaching down and out with your right arm while your left elbow bends upward as far as it can go. You should feel a pull up the left side of your body. Let your head relax to the right. Keep your left shoulder back and your hips forward.

3. Come back up almost into the starting position. This down-and-up movement is done to one count. Do 10 to 20 counts to the right and then repeat to the left.

APRIL

	MORNING	AFTERNOON
9 MONDAY		
10 TUESDAY		
11 WEDNESDAY		
12 THURSDAY		
13 FRIDAY		
14 SATURDAY		
15 SUNDAY	PALM SUNDAY	

Exercise—Waist
Health Challenge—Cut Down on Sugar

OPEN STRIDE
FLOOR STRETCH

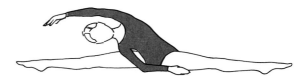

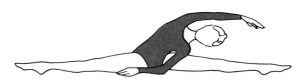

Sit on the floor with your legs as far apart as you can without feeling strained, keeping the backs of your knees pressed into the floor. Toes pointed. Lengthen your torso out of your hips and then reach to the right with the left arm overhead, keeping both hips on the floor and legs turned out. Reach as far to the right as you can, arm over the ear. Hold the stretch, breathe, return to the center and repeat to the other side. Continue the exercise until you have felt a good stretch.

APRIL

	MORNING	AFTERNOON
16 MONDAY		
17 TUESDAY	PASSOVER, FIRST DAY	
18 WEDNESDAY		
19 THURSDAY		
20 FRIDAY	GOOD FRIDAY	
21 SATURDAY		
22 SUNDAY	EASTER	

Exercise—Waist
Health Challenge—Cut Down on Sugar

STANDING WAIST STRETCH

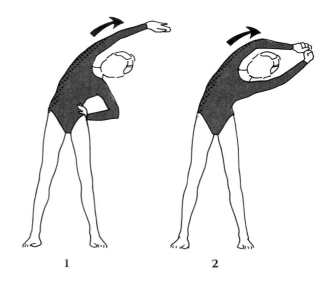

1   2

1. Stand with your feet a little more than hip-distance apart. With your left hand on your hip, reach your right hand over your head and slowly bend at your waist to the left side. Hold, breathe, feel a good stretch. Return to center and repeat to the other side.

2. The next time you stretch to the side, instead of putting your hand on your hip, grab your right hand with your left hand and then bend slowly to the left, keeping your hips forward and your shoulders facing front. Hold the stretch, breathe, relax, return to center and repeat to the other side. Try to increase the time you hold each stretch. *Do not bounce.* Repeat until you feel well stretched.

APRIL

	MORNING	AFTERNOON
23 MONDAY		
24 TUESDAY		
25 WEDNESDAY		
26 THURSDAY		
27 FRIDAY		
28 SATURDAY		
29 SUNDAY		

Exercise—Waist
Health Challenge—Cut Down on Sugar

My Protein Drink

I have a low-calorie, filling protein drink that will satisfy your sweet tooth. It's my basic breakfast. I give no amounts here. Use your judgment and go by taste. It should be thick and delicious. In your blender, put non-fat milk, apple juice (that's the sweetener—make it organic if possible), fresh frozen strawberries or peaches (not the kind in syrup), half a papaya, half a banana (a whole one if weight's no problem), and protein powder. Then blend it all until smooth and thick. If you have no frozen fruit, use fresh fruit and add several ice cubes.

When buying a protein powder, look for one that contains no sugar, preservatives, artificial colorings or flavor. The powder I use is made from milk and egg protein, which I believe is easier to digest and absorb than powders made from soya protein.

Baked Indian Pudding

1 *quart milk*
⅓ *cup cornmeal*
2 *tablespoons soy flour*
⅓ *cup sweet cider*
½ *teaspoon salt*
½ *teaspoon cinnamon, ground*
½ *teaspoon ginger, ground*
½ *cup molasses*
3 *tablespoons nutritional yeast (optional)*
½ *cup dried fruit, chopped (optional)*

Scald milk in top of double boiler over direct heat. Make paste of cornmeal and soy flour in cider. Blend with milk, cover and cook over hot water for 20 minutes. Add rest of ingredients. Remove from heat. Turn into oiled casserole. Bake at 325° for 2 hours or until set. Serve hot, topped with yogurt. Serves 6.

APRIL/MAY

	MORNING	AFTERNOON
30 MONDAY		
1 TUESDAY		
2 WEDNESDAY		
3 THURSDAY		
4 FRIDAY		
5 SATURDAY		
6 SUNDAY		

Exercise—Waist
Health Challenge—Cut Down on Sugar

Strawberry Sponge

1 *cup boiling water*
1 *package strawberry gelatin*
¾ *cup cold water*
½ *cup chilled evaporated milk*
2 *tablespoons lemon juice*
¼ *cup powdered milk*

Combine boiling water with gelatin and stir well. Add cold water and chill until gelatin starts to congeal. Meanwhile beat evaporated milk until it stiffens, then add lemon juice and powdered milk and beat together slightly. Fold whipped milk into gelatin with 1 cup sliced and sweetened fresh or frozen strawberries. Pour into mold and chill until set.

VARIATIONS:

- Omit strawberries from sponge; pour sponge into ring mold; unmold and fill center with sliced and sweetened or frozen strawberries.
- Use raspberry gelatin; fold in fresh or frozen raspberries.
- Use lemon gelatin; fold in 1 cup mashed banana.
- Use lime gelatin; fold in 1 cup well-drained pineapple; use juice from pineapple instead of part of the cold water.
- Use orange gelatin; add grated rind of 1 orange and/or 1 teaspoon orange flavoring; fill center of ring mold with sweetened orange sections.
- Yogurt sponge: Omit evaporated milk and lemon juice; fold into gelatin 1 cup thick yogurt; prepare as in basic recipe or any variation. Yogurt is particularly delicious in the lime-pineapple combination.
- Gelatin chiffon pies: Prepare basic recipe or any variation; pour into a 9-inch pie plate brushed with soft margarine or butter and sprinkled with cereal, cracker, or cookie crumbs; sprinkle top with crumbs.
- Lemon sponge: Use lemon gelatin; instead of ½ cup water, cool with ½ cup lemon juice; sprinkle buttered square mold or 9-inch pie plate with cereal, cookie, or cracker crumbs; pour gelatin over crumbs and sprinkle top with crumbs; chill; cut into cubes or wedges and serve.

MAY

S	M	T	W	T	F	S
		1	2	3	4	5
6	7	8	9	10	11	12
13	14	15	16	17	18	19
20	21	22	23	24	25	26
27	28	29	30	31		

EXERCISE—
ABDOMINALS

Abdominal Stretch
Bent-Knee Sit-ups
Abdominal Curl

HEALTH CHALLENGE—
EAT MORE FRESH VEGETABLES

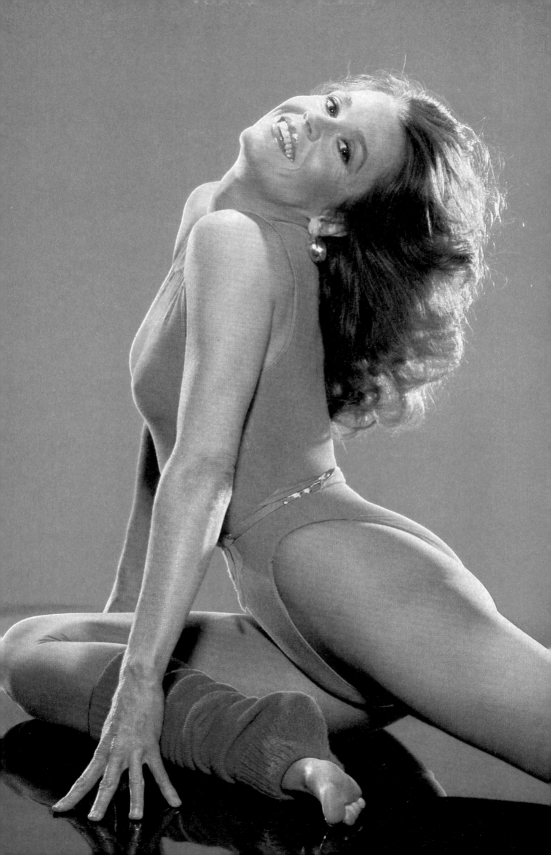

Exercise—ABDOMINALS

Strong abdominal muscles are the best insurance against lower back pain. They help the back muscles to support the spinal column by holding the abdominal organs in, pressed up against the spine where the spine tends to be weakest—in the lower back (lumbar) area.

When doing these abdominal exercises, *never allow your back to arch.* Keep pressing the lower back into the floor.

Health Challenge—EAT MORE FRESH VEGETABLES

A general rule of thumb for healthful eating is: *Eat food that is as close to its natural, living state as possible.*

Fresh vegetables should make up a major portion of your daily diet. They contain complex carbohydrates which provide more sustained energy over a greater length of time than simple carbohydrates.

Vegetables are high in fiber, which is vital for healthy intestines and helps regulate the bowels, thereby reducing the risk of intestinal and rectal cancer. High-fiber foods are digested slowly, which means that their glucose enters the system at a slow rate and gives us a steady, long-term supply of energy. Fiber is also important for people who want to lose weight, because it decreases the amount of calories you absorb from your food. These are some of the reasons, in addition to all the vitamins they provide, why you should eat a lot of fresh vegetables.

There are many delicious ways to eat vegetables raw, which is the best way to get the most nutritional punch from your meal.

If you cook your vegetables, the best way is to steam them. Put the vegetables in a steamer basket inside a pot containing boiling water. The water should not touch the vegetables. Cover the pot and steam until the vegetables are "al dente" or crunchy. Never cook them so long they become soggy. Overcooking and soaking in water causes vegetables to lose much of their nutritional value.

APRIL/MAY

	MORNING		AFTERNOON
30 MONDAY			
1 TUESDAY			
2 WEDNESDAY			
3 THURSDAY			
4 FRIDAY			
5 SATURDAY			
6 SUNDAY			

Exercise—Abdominals
Health Challenge—Eat More Fresh Vegetables

ABDOMINAL STRETCH

Lie on your back with your legs out straight and your arms extended on the floor over your head. Stretch the right arm and right leg out from the body in opposite directions, feeling a stretch up the right side. Hold for eight seconds, release and then repeat to the left. Don't let the lower back arch.

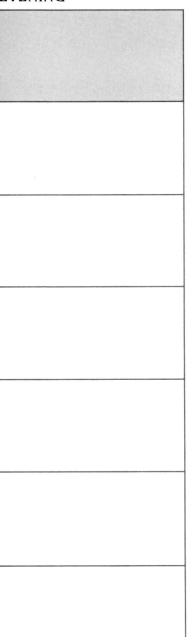

MAY

	MORNING	AFTERNOON
7 MONDAY		
8 TUESDAY		
9 WEDNESDAY		
10 THURSDAY		
11 FRIDAY		
12 SATURDAY		
13 SUNDAY	MOTHER'S DAY	

Exercise—Abdominals
Health Challenge—Eat More Fresh Vegetables

BENT-KNEE SIT-UPS

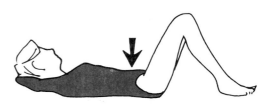

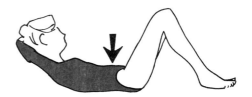

Lie down with your knees bent, feet a little more than hip-distance apart, toes and knees parallel, hands clasped behind your head with elbows back, chin up. Contract your stomach muscles by pushing the lower back into the floor, then lift your upper body several inches. Hold a second and release slightly but don't lower all the way to the floor; then lift again. Exhale as you lift, inhale as you release. Do as many times as you can in a steady, rhythmic tempo.

There are several things to bear in mind when doing these Bent-Knee Sit-ups:

1. Your head and neck should be relaxed. Don't hold your head up with the neck but let your hands and arms support it.
2. Don't tuck your chin in; look up at the ceiling, not at your knees.
3. Keep your elbows back.
4. Don't use your arms to lift your upper body. You lift by contracting inward. Think of pushing a penny into the floor with your lower back. Another image that might help is to think of someone punching you in the stomach, causing you to contract inward while your upper body lifts.

MAY

	MORNING	AFTERNOON
14 MONDAY		
15 TUESDAY		
16 WEDNESDAY		
17 THURSDAY		
18 FRIDAY		
19 SATURDAY		
20 SUNDAY		

Exercise—Abdominals
Health Challenge—Eat More Fresh Vegetables

ABDOMINAL CURL

Lie on your back with knees bent and lifted toward your chest. Clasp your hands behind your head and, keeping your chin tucked in and elbows forward alongside your ears, lift your head and shoulders until your elbows touch your knees. Release slightly (don't let your head and shoulders touch the floor) and lift again. Exhale as you lift, inhale as you release. Repeat as many times as you can in a steady, rhythmic tempo.

MAY

	MORNING	AFTERNOON
21 MONDAY		
22 TUESDAY		
23 WEDNESDAY		
24 THURSDAY		
25 FRIDAY		
26 SATURDAY		
27 SUNDAY		

Exercise—Abdominals
Health Challenge—Eat More Fresh Vegetables

My One-Meal Salad

Cut in small pieces each of the vegetables you like the most. A good combination is zucchini or yellow squash, radishes, carrots, cucumber, celery, apple, cauliflower, jicama, onions, green pepper and fresh mushrooms. Make a good low-cal dressing, then put a little grated cheese, nuts or sunflower seeds on top and you are ready to go!

Cucumber Boats

Cut a cucumber in half lengthwise and, without puncturing the skin, take out the inside and chop fine. Mix with plain yogurt and finely chopped onions, fill the "boats" with the mixture, and chill. Put some chopped radishes on top to garnish. You won't believe the taste! Serves 1 or 2.

Gazpacho Salad

1 *clove garlic*
4 *whole tomatoes*
½ *small onion*
½ *green pepper*
1 *whole cucumber*
¼ *tablespoon freshly ground pepper*
2 *tablespoons sunflower seed oil*
3 *tablespoons vinegar*
½ *cup water*
Oregano, marjoram or basil to taste

To make this the old Spanish way you hand-chop all the vegetables fine and mix with the remaining ingredients, but you can use the blender for a couple of seconds instead. Serve cold in soup bowls and sprinkle some of the cut up vegetables on top. Serves 2 or 3.

MAY/JUNE

	MORNING	AFTERNOON
28 MONDAY	MEMORIAL DAY OBSERVED	
29 TUESDAY		
30 WEDNESDAY	MEMORIAL DAY	
31 THURSDAY		
1 FRIDAY		
2 SATURDAY		
3 SUNDAY		

Exercise—Abdominals
Health Challenge—Eat More Fresh Vegetables

Lemon-Sesame Dressing

½ cup lemon juice
2 tablespoons tamari soy sauce
2 tablespoons water
¼ cup plus 2 tablespoons oil
¼ cup tahini
¼ teaspoon garlic powder
¼ teaspoon celery seeds
¼ green pepper, chopped
¼ cup sliced onions

Combine all ingredients in electric blender and process until smooth. Makes 2 cups.

Curried Broccoli and Carrots

2 medium-size onions, sliced
2 cloves garlic, minced
¼ cup oil
½ teaspoon turmeric
1 teaspoon ground coriander
1 teaspoon ground cumin
½ pound carrots (approximately 2 carrots)
1 pound broccoli (approximately ½ of large bunch)
⅛ teaspoon chili powder or crushed dried chili peppers
½ cup water, more if needed

Sauté onions and garlic in oil for a few minutes, stir in turmeric, coriander and cumin, then add carrots. Cover pan, turn down heat and steam for 5 minutes. Add broccoli, then chili powder and finally add the water. Cover pan again and cook over low heat for another 10 minutes or until vegetables are tender but still firm. Serves 4 to 6.

JUNE

S	M	T	W	T	F	S
					1	2
3	4	5	6	7	8	9
10	11	12	13	14	15	16
17	18	19	20	21	22	23
24	25	26	27	28	29	30

EXERCISE—
BACK

Lower Back and Hip Stretch
Lower Back Stretch
Back Stretch
Squat

HEALTH CHALLENGE—
EAT MORE FRESH FRUIT

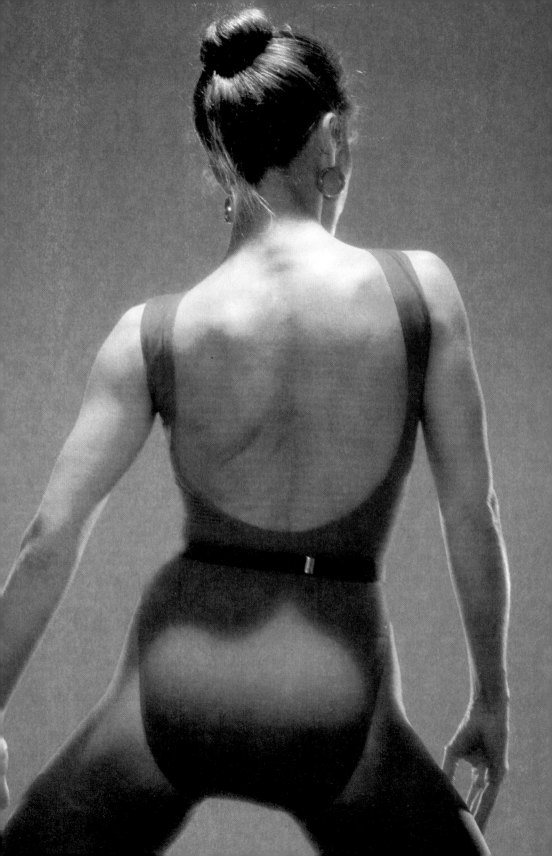

JUNE

Exercise—BACK

Seven million people in the U.S. suffer from back pain. Two million of them cannot work as a result. Seventy-five percent of people with back pain are obese; obesity causes a weak and protruding abdomen and swayback, which puts pressure on the lumbar region (the lower back). Other causes of back pain include poor posture and psychological stress. Under stress, people tense their muscles, which can cause the muscles to go into spasm. Spasms, in turn, restrict blood circulation to the muscles involved, which, if already weak, can become painful.

Only ten percent of back pain is caused by actual structural defects. It is generally agreed now that exercise is the best way to prevent back pain and to strengthen a back that has already given you problems. Exercise helps to reduce weight, strengthens supportive muscles and increases circulation of nutrient-carrying blood to the spine.

Good activities for people with back problems are walking, swimming (crawl and back stroke), cross-country skiing and cycling in an upright position.

There are other indoor exercises which are excellent for the back and a number of critical dos and don'ts:

1. Be conscious of standing tall, pulling up out of your torso, holding your stomach in.
2. If you must stand for long periods of time, place one foot on a stool or footrest approximately four to six inches off the floor. This relieves swayback and the resultant pressure on the lower back.
3. Don't wear high heels all the time. They shorten the Achilles' tendon (the tendon between the heel and the calf muscle) and put pressure on the soft tissues in the lower back.
4. When lifting heavy objects, keep your knees bent and your back straight. Use your arm and leg muscles to do the work.
5. Never lift heavy objects over your head, which causes the back to arch.

6. Avoid prolonged sitting. Get up and stretch and walk around every hour.
7. When sitting, your knees should be higher than your hips when your feet are flat on the ground. Short people when sitting should put a low stool under their feet if their knees drop below their hips or dangle in the air.
8. Never use a chair that sticks into the small of your back. The back of the chair should be firm, giving flat support to the upper lumbar region.
9. Sleep in a firm bed. If your mattress is soft, put a three-quarter-inch plywood board under it. A thinner board will not be solid enough.

If you have had a back injury, have a chronic defect or are experiencing prolonged back pain, you will need more specific instruction from a qualified professional—and remember: If an exercise causes pain in your back, *don't do it!*

Health Challenge—EAT MORE FRESH FRUIT

Let delicious, cold, sweet, fresh fruit replace candy in your life. Learn to savor the sweetness. Discover how fresh fruit can be an energy booster. The energy you get from sugar, while it does give you a quick jolt, triggers an insulin reaction that causes a precipitous drop in blood sugar, leaving you feeling quickly tired—and craving more sweets. Complex foods like fruit, vegetables, and grains, on the other hand, break down into glucose more slowly, which means that the energy they provide will be more sustained. If you are trying to lose weight, limit yourself to three pieces of fresh fruit a day to avoid overdoing the natural fruit sugar.

MAY/JUNE

	MORNING	AFTERNOON
28 MONDAY		
29 TUESDAY		
30 WEDNESDAY		
31 THURSDAY		
1 FRIDAY		
2 SATURDAY		
3 SUNDAY		

Exercise—Back
Health Challenge—Eat More Fresh Fruit

LOWER BACK AND
HIP STRETCH

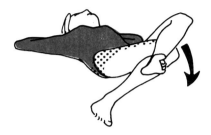

Lie down, place your feet flat on the floor and your hands behind your head, elbows resting on the floor. Cross your left leg over your right leg. Let the weight of your left leg press your right leg as far over to the left as you can, keeping your elbows, shoulders and upper back flat on the floor. Stretch, breathe, and don't tense. Hold for forty seconds, then release. Repeat to the other side, with the right leg crossed over the left leg and pressing down to the right.

JUNE

	MORNING	AFTERNOON
4 MONDAY		
5 TUESDAY		
6 WEDNESDAY		
7 THURSDAY		
8 FRIDAY		
9 SATURDAY		
10 SUNDAY		

Exercise—Back
Health Challenge—Eat More Fresh Fruit

LOWER BACK STRETCH

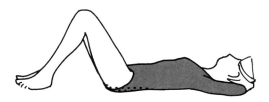

   Lying on your back with knees bent, feet flat on the floor a little more than hip-distance apart and hands behind your head, squeeze your buttocks as you push your lower back into the floor and tighten your abdominal muscles. Hold this contraction ten seconds, release and repeat again a number of times.

BACK STRETCH

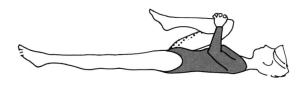

   Lie flat on your back with legs straight. Bend your right knee, grasp with both hands and gently pull it toward your chest, keeping the back of your neck pressed into the floor. Hold for forty seconds. Lower the leg and repeat with the left one.

JUNE

	MORNING	AFTERNOON
11 MONDAY		
12 TUESDAY		
13 WEDNESDAY		
14 THURSDAY		
15 FRIDAY		
16 SATURDAY		
17 SUNDAY	FATHER'S DAY	

Exercise—Back
Health Challenge—Eat More Fresh Fruit

SQUAT

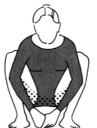

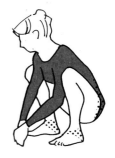

Squat with your feet flat and slightly turned out, heels about one foot apart. Arms should be inside the knees, putting gentle pressure on the knees to keep them from rolling in. Knees should be directly above the toes. Hold for as long as is comfortable.

JUNE

	MORNING	AFTERNOON
18 MONDAY		
19 TUESDAY		
20 WEDNESDAY		
21 THURSDAY		
22 FRIDAY		
23 SATURDAY		
24 SUNDAY		

Exercise—Back
Health Challenge—Eat More Fresh Fruit

Fruit Salad

Good Fruit Combinations:
1. Mix three different kinds of melons.
2. Peaches, plums, cherries.
3. Bananas, grapes, strawberries.

Put slices of sweet honeydew in the freezer for a delicious fruit popsicle.

Yam-Fruit Salad

5 *yams, cooked and diced*
4 *bananas, sliced*
3 *apples with skins, diced*
1 *cup seedless grapes*

Lightly toss all ingredients. Moisten with favorite dressing. Serves 6.

Salad of India

6 *bananas, sliced*
3 *tablespoons mint, minced*
½ *cup dates, pitted and chopped*
½ *cup nuts, ground*

Arrange banana slices on bed of greens. Garnish with the other ingredients. Serves 6.

Suggested combination fruit salads:
Pineapple, grapefruit, bananas, alfalfa sprouts
Apple, celery, pear, fenugreek sprouts
Banana, apple, raisins, coconut shreds

JUNE/JULY

	MORNING	AFTERNOON
25 MONDAY		
26 TUESDAY		
27 WEDNESDAY		
28 THURSDAY		
29 FRIDAY		
30 SATURDAY		
1 SUNDAY		

Exercise—Back
Health Challenge—Eat More Fresh Fruit

Papaya à la Ashram

Cut a ripe papaya in half and remove the seeds. Mix fresh chopped mushrooms, sunflower seeds, low-cal mayonnaise and/or yogurt together, season with curry powder, fill the papaya and sprinkle dill weed on top. Serve chilled on a bed of lettuce. As a variation use crabmeat. How beautiful!

Fruit Salad Dressing

Mix equal parts of yogurt and ricotta cheese in a blender. Add your favorite juice—orange, pineapple, strawberry or apple, then add any flavor you like—vanilla, banana, almond. Top off with cinnamon, then pour over your fruit salad and ENJOY!

JULY

S	M	T	W	T	F	S
1	2	3	4	5	6	7
8	9	10	11	12	13	14
15	16	17	18	19	20	21
22	23	24	25	26	27	28
29	30	31				

EXERCISE—
HIPS AND UPPER THIGHS

Hip Stretch
Lower Back and Hip Stretch
Back of Hips
Crossovers

HEALTH CHALLENGE—
EAT LESS MEAT

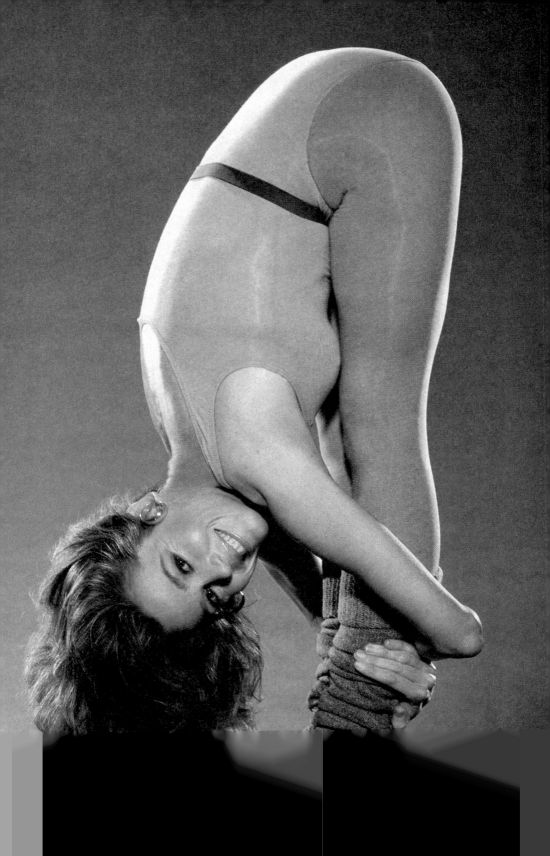

JULY

Exercise—HIPS AND UPPER THIGHS

Nice, rounded hips are beautiful. But because of the normal tendency for women to have extra layers of fat on their hips and thighs, and the difficulty of developing muscle tone in that area without specific exercise, the metabolism in the hip and thigh tends to be sluggish. Fat, unlike muscle, is an inactive tissue and burns few calories. Hence, without proper exercise the lovely round hips and thighs become "saddlebags." Eating a lot of salty, sugary, processed foods compounds the problem.

Basic rules for the elimination of saddlebags: Cut out salt; reduce sugar and fat; drink *lots* of water; and *exercise.*

I've given some of the best hip exercises here. They will strengthen and increase the muscle tone in the hips, which means the metabolism will also improve. But the best way to reduce fatty deposits is to combine these localized exercises with increasing amounts of aerobic movement to burn calories; so keep up the jogging, Jumping Jacks, walking, and Step-ups. Remember, you're trying to work up to fifteen to thirty minutes of aerobics a day, three to five times a week.

Health Challenge—EAT LESS MEAT

Most of us were brought up believing that we need large amounts of protein and that the best way to get it is to eat lots of meat. Protein is important for the body's chemical reactions, but research has now shown that we eat much more protein than we really need. Thirty to fifty grams of protein a day is ample.

Certain people, under particular circumstances, may need more, such as athletes, pregnant or breast-feeding women, and people fighting off infections. Or, if you are cutting way down on your intake of calories, some of the protein you are consuming may be used up to provide the energy that you normally get from carbohydrates, and this may mean you are not getting enough protein to meet your body's needs. Also don't cut back on protein during times of stress, when the body's need for protein increases.

We will do our bodies the greatest good if we get most of our protein from vegetable rather than animal sources. Ninety percent of the meat we buy contains antibiotics, synthetic hormones, and other chemicals which are fed to livestock to stimulate growth, combat disease, and force weight gain. Their residues are often found in animal tissues and are not eliminated through cooking. These can cause allergic reactions, upset the gastrointestinal processes and build up immunities to certain life-saving drugs.

In addition, most livestock are raised in feed lots and their fat is entirely *saturated*. Saturated fat increases the cholesterol level in the blood and the danger of heart disease. A major advantage to getting your protein from vegetable sources like beans and rice is that they are cholesterol-free. You don't need meat as your source of protein as long as you eat enough fresh, natural plant protein such as is found in beans, brown rice, and cereals, and non-meat protein like milk, cheese and eggs.

If you want to lose weight you can get your needed protein with fewer calories and less fat by eating broiled fish (the best, healthiest source of animal protein) and the white meat of chicken with the skin removed.

So, this month, see if you can go without eating meat—any kind of meat. I'm not advocating that you become a permanent vegetarian (though *informed* vegetarians probably eat the most healthful diet) but perhaps, after a meatless month, you will discover that it's not all that difficult to cut way back.

A special note to women who are developing wrinkles: After a month without meat see if you don't notice a lessening of the lines and puffiness around your eyes—it's the reduction in fat that does it. You'll take that a step further next month.

JULY

	MORNING	AFTERNOON
1 SUNDAY 2 MONDAY		
3 TUESDAY		
4 WEDNESDAY	INDEPENDENCE DAY	
5 THURSDAY		
6 FRIDAY		
7 SATURDAY		
8 SUNDAY		

Exercise—Hips and Upper Thighs
Health Challenge—Eat Less Meat

HIP STRETCH

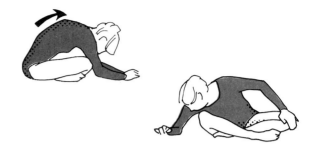

Sit up straight with your legs crossed, right leg in front of your left. Now round your back down over your legs until you feel a good stretch in your back and hips. Try to place your elbows on the floor in front of you. Now round your back down over the right knee until you feel a good stretch, breathe, hold, release and sit up. Recross your legs so the left leg is in front. Repeat, rounding down in front then to the side over your left knee.

LOWER BACK AND HIP STRETCH

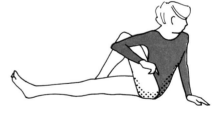

Sit with your right leg straight ahead and flat on the floor. Bend your left leg, cross your left foot over and place it down flat outside your right knee. Bend your right elbow and rest it on the outside of your upper left thigh just below the knee. Place your left hand behind you and slowly turn your head and upper body to look over your left shoulder. As you do this, gently press your right elbow in the opposite direction against your left thigh. Hold, breathe easily, repeat to the other side.

JULY

	MORNING	AFTERNOON
9 MONDAY		
10 TUESDAY		
11 WEDNESDAY		
12 THURSDAY		
13 FRIDAY		
14 SATURDAY		
15 SUNDAY		

Exercise—Hips and Upper Thighs
Health Challenge—Eat Less Meat

BACK OF HIPS

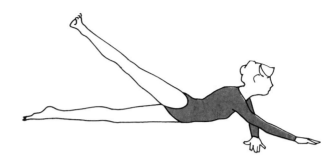

Lie on your stomach, raise your head and chest off the floor and support yourself on your elbows. Lift your right leg as high as you can, then lower it several inches, but without touching the floor. This is a small movement, lifting from a lifted position. Concentrate on working the back of the hip. Continue this lift until your hip muscle tires. Then repeat with the left leg. This exercise also strengthens muscles of the back. If you have any history of back problems or are over fifty, do this exercise with your chest on the floor.

JULY

	MORNING	AFTERNOON
16 MONDAY		
17 TUESDAY		
18 WEDNESDAY		
19 THURSDAY		
20 FRIDAY		
21 SATURDAY		
22 SUNDAY		

Exercise—Hips and Upper Thighs
Health Challenge—Eat Less Meat

CROSSOVERS

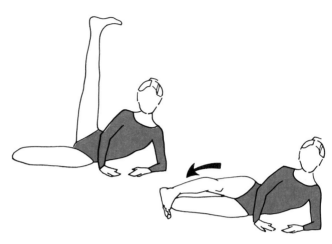

Lie on your left side with your head and torso raised and supported by your left elbow. Flex the left knee so that the thigh is in a line with your torso and raise the right leg straight up with the foot flexed. Keeping your hips still and your knees straight, lower your leg in front of you at a comfortable angle to about three inches above the floor, then lift it up again. Continue this movement with a steady rhythm until the hip muscle tires. Then repeat to the other side. It is important when lifting the leg not to let your hips rock backward to help you. Imagine there is a wall behind your hips pressing them forward and a friend is pulling your right foot away from your body as you lower your leg. It is stretched so far out from your body that you need your right hand on the floor in front of you for balance. Inhale as you lower your leg, exhale as you raise it.

JULY

	MORNING	AFTERNOON
23 MONDAY		
24 TUESDAY		
25 WEDNESDAY		
26 THURSDAY		
27 FRIDAY		
28 SATURDAY		
29 SUNDAY		

Exercise—Hips and Upper Thighs
Health Challenge—Eat Less Meat

Xergis

3 cucumbers
1 onion
1 small clove garlic or dash garlic powder
5 cups yogurt
1 teaspoon oil
4 teaspoons dill weed
Dash pepper

Peel cucumbers and remove seeds. Chop the cucumbers, onion, and garlic fine. Put in blender with half the yogurt, the oil, dill weed, salt, and pepper. Blend. Pour out some of the mixture, add remaining yogurt, and blend again. Combine and chill. Serves 6.

Baked Fish

2 pounds fish of your choice (fresh or fresh frozen)
2 tablespoons lemon juice (fresh)
3 tablespoons chopped parsley
1/4 cup chopped chives
2 tablespoons dill weed
1/4 cup chopped onion
1/4 cup chopped celery

Preheat oven to 325°. Rinse fish; allow to drain. Place fish in oiled baking dish. Mix together all remaining ingredients and sprinkle on fish. Cover dish with foil, sealing the edges. Bake 20 minutes at 325°. Fish is done when it flakes easily with a fork. Remove to a hot platter. Garnish with lemon slices and parsley. Serves 4.

Here's an extra tip: Use the cold left-over fish chopped up over a tossed salad.

JULY/AUGUST

	MORNING	AFTERNOON
30 MONDAY		
31 TUESDAY		
1 WEDNESDAY		
2 THURSDAY		
3 FRIDAY		
4 SATURDAY		
5 SUNDAY		

Exercise—Hips and Upper Thighs
Health Challenge—Eat Less Meat

Soy Burgers

2 tablespoons oil
2 tablespoons chopped green onions
1 cup cooked soy pulp, or coarsely chopped
   soybeans
1 cup cooked brown rice
½ cup grated cheese
1 cup toasted sesame and/or sunflower seeds,
   ground
⅓ cup whole wheat flour
2 eggs, beaten
2 teaspoons soy sauce
½ teaspoon basil

Sauté onions in oil and mix into remaining ingredients. Shape into patties and cook on a griddle or in a skillet. You can also bake patties in a 350° oven for 20 minutes. To keep them from sticking, sprinkle griddle or baking dish with sesame seeds. Makes 8.

AUGUST

S	M	T	W	T	F	S
			1	2	3	4
5	6	7	8	9	10	11
12	13	14	15	16	17	18
19	20	21	22	23	24	25
26	27	28	29	30	31	

EXERCISE—
INNER THIGHS

Standing Stretch
Groin and Hamstring Stretch
Standing Leg and Hip Stretch
Inner Thigh Lift

HEALTH CHALLENGE—
REDUCE INTAKE OF FAT

112

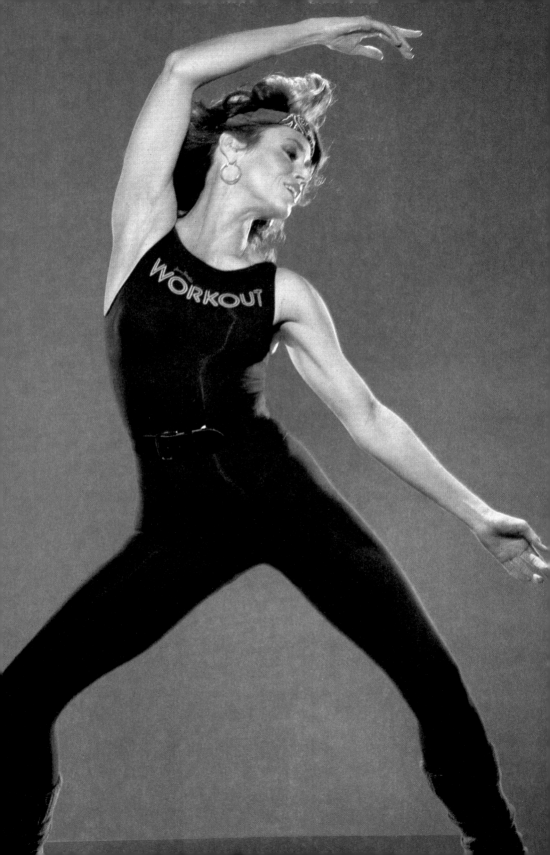

AUGUST

Exercise—INNER THIGHS

Inner thighs are another area where women tend to develop fatty deposits. Most sports do not develop muscle tone and firmness in that area, hence the wibble-wobbles that begin to appear along the inside of the thighs after a certain age. The following exercises are the best way to isolate that area in order to improve muscle tone and increase metabolism.

Health Challenge—REDUCE INTAKE OF FAT

More than forty percent of the average American diet is composed of fat. Fat, of course, is essential. Vitamins A, D, K and E are available to the body only in combination with fats. Fat also provides necessary fatty acids. But by eating vegetables and grains, we get all the fat we need. We do not need animal fats or other oils.

You've already cut way down on one major source of fat—meat. This month, you'll try to go even further. This is important because fat supplies more than twice as many calories as proteins and carbohydrates do (nine calories per gram) and as I've already pointed out, saturated animal fats such as butter, lard, and shortening, which are solid at room temperature, increase the cholesterol level and are dangerous for the heart. In addition, fats limit the amount of oxygen which can get to the cells in the body. Oxygen is essential to preventing the development of atherosclerosis.

If you must use fat for cooking, it is preferable to use a cold-pressed, unsaturated oil (liquid at room temperature). Vegetable oils like corn and safflower oil are examples. Since vegetable oils become rancid very quickly, it is best to buy them in small amounts and keep them refrigerated. Two vegetable oils to *avoid* are peanut and coconut oil.

Other ways to reduce fat:
1. Use non-fat instead of whole milk.
2. Eat farmer's cheese, low-fat cottage cheese, feta and mozzarella instead of high-fat cheese.
3. Substitute low-fat yogurt for sour cream.
4. If you go back to eating meats now and then, buy lean cuts and trim off all the excess fat.

JULY/AUGUST

	MORNING	AFTERNOON
30 MONDAY		
31 TUESDAY		
1 WEDNESDAY		
2 THURSDAY		
3 FRIDAY		
4 SATURDAY		
5 SUNDAY		

Exercise—Inner Thighs
Health Challenge—Reduce Intake of Fat

STANDING STRETCH

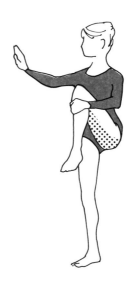

Stand on one leg with your hand resting on something for support. Grasp your knee with the other hand and pull it to your chest while keeping your back straight and your hips under. Bend your standing leg slightly and point your toes straight ahead. Hold, then repeat to the other side.

AUGUST

	MORNING	AFTERNOON
6 MONDAY		
7 TUESDAY		
8 WEDNESDAY		
9 THURSDAY		
10 FRIDAY		
11 SATURDAY		
12 SUNDAY		

Exercise—Inner Thighs
Health Challenge—Reduce Intake of Fat

GROIN AND HAMSTRING STRETCH

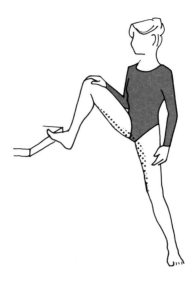

Stand and place the toes of one foot on something solid about table height with your heel stretching down. Hold on to something for balance, if necessary. Turn the foot of the standing leg out, parallel to the support. Then bend your raised knee as you press your hips forward as far as you can without tensing. Hold, release. Repeat and then do the same thing to the other side.

AUGUST

	MORNING	AFTERNOON
13 MONDAY		
14 TUESDAY		
15 WEDNESDAY		
16 THURSDAY		
17 FRIDAY		
18 SATURDAY		
19 SUNDAY		

Exercise—Inner Thighs
Health Challenge—Reduce Intake of Fat

STANDING LEG AND HIP STRETCH

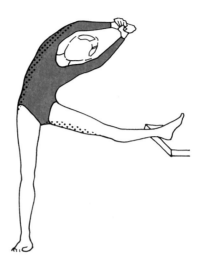

Place your left leg on something solid about table height. Turn the foot of the right leg so that it is parallel to the support and turn your body to face that same direction. Grasp your right wrist with your left hand and as though you were pulling your right hand and arm up and over your head, slowly bend sideways toward the raised leg, keep your upper body facing straight ahead. Hold the stretch and release slowly. Repeat with opposite leg.

AUGUST

	MORNING	AFTERNOON
20 MONDAY		
21 TUESDAY		
22 WEDNESDAY		
23 THURSDAY		
24 FRIDAY		
25 SATURDAY		
26 SUNDAY		

Exercise—Inner Thighs
Health Challenge—Reduce Intake of Fat

INNER THIGH LIFT

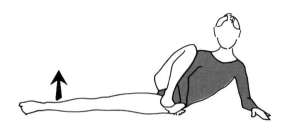

Lie on your left side, supported on your left elbow, your body in a straight line with your left leg. Cross your right leg over the left and place your toes on the floor and your right hand on the right foot. Be very sure the bottom leg is turned out with the inner thigh facing the ceiling. When you look down at your leg, you should see your inner thigh, not the top of your leg. Your weight should be directly on the left hip. Keeping your toes pointed, lift the left leg up several inches above the floor and then lower it again without touching the floor. Repeat 10 to 20 times. Pause, flex your left foot, move it backward three inches and lift-lower again 10 to 20 times. Repeat to the other side.

AUGUST/SEPTEMBER

	MORNING	AFTERNOON
27 MONDAY		
28 TUESDAY		
29 WEDNESDAY		
30 THURSDAY		
31 FRIDAY		
1 SATURDAY		
2 SUNDAY		

Exercise—Inner Thighs
Health Challenge—Reduce Intake of Fat

Creamy Yogurt-Garlic Dressing

¾ cup plain yogurt
1 tablespoon mayonnaise (or oil)
1 or 2 cloves garlic, pressed
Pepper to taste (or kelp and cayenne)

Combine all ingredients in blender and whiz until smooth. (18 calories/tablespoon)

VARIATIONS:
Add chopped vegetables or herbs to the dressing, such as:

1 scallion
2 tablespoons fresh parsley
½ teaspoon each basil and oregano
Fresh or dried dill to taste
1 ounce firmly crumbled blue or Roquefort cheese

Red Lotus

Scoop out the inside of a tomato. Chop the pulp and mix with cottage cheese, chopped green apple, green onion, green pepper, jicama (if available), and celery. Add spices to taste and fill tomato. Low in calories but high in food value.

SEPTEMBER

S	M	T	W	T	F	S
						1
2	3	4	5	6	7	8
9	10	11	12	13	14	15
16	17	18	19	20	21	22
23	24	25	26	27	28	29
30						

EXERCISE—
BUTTOCKS

Buttocks Stretch
Buttocks Lift
Groin and Hip Stretch

HEALTH CHALLENGE—
ELIMINATE PROCESSED FOODS

126

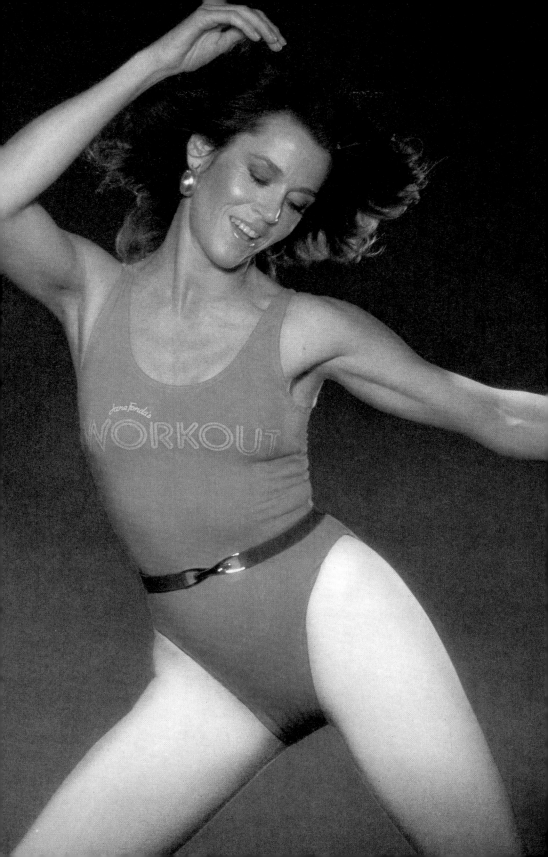

SEPTEMBER

Exercise—BUTTOCKS

These buttocks exercises are excellent for women who tend to be flat-butted and want to build a nice round muscle back there. And for those of us who carry around a large posterior, remember: if it's big, make it high, round and hard!—and these exercises will do it.

Health Challenge—ELIMINATE PROCESSED FOODS

Processed food tends to be high in salt and sugar and low in nutritional value. The process of milling, refining, flaking, puffing and preserving destroys many of the essential vitamins, minerals and trace elements. Few of these are replaced by "enriching."

In addition, processed foods often contain chemical additives which can cause allergic reactions, upset the delicate chemical balances within the body and impede the absorption of essential vitamins and minerals. Hyperactivity and learning disabilities in some children have been linked to food colorings and flavorings.

Make a habit of reading food labels before you buy. Avoid products that contain such questionable additives as nitrates, saccharin, sodium, artificial colorings and petroleum additives such as BHA and BHT.

This month, try to junk the junk food entirely and stick to foods that are as close to their natural, living or growing state as possible.

AUGUST/SEPTEMBER

	MORNING	AFTERNOON
27 MONDAY		
28 TUESDAY		
29 WEDNESDAY		
30 THURSDAY		
31 FRIDAY		
1 SATURDAY		
2 SUNDAY		

Exercise—Buttocks
Health Challenge—Eliminate Processed Foods

BUTTOCKS STRETCH

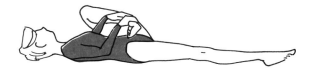

    Lying on your back with legs straight, flex your left knee, grab your left foot with both hands, and stretch it across your groin until you feel a good stretch in the left hip. Repeat to the other side.

SEPTEMBER

	MORNING	AFTERNOON
3 MONDAY	LABOR DAY	
4 TUESDAY		
5 WEDNESDAY		
6 THURSDAY		
7 FRIDAY		
8 SATURDAY		
9 SUNDAY		

Exercise—Buttocks
Health Challenge—Eliminate Processed Foods

BUTTOCKS LIFT

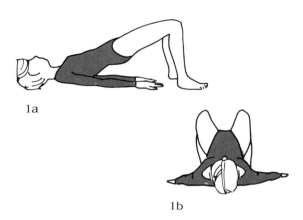

1a

1b

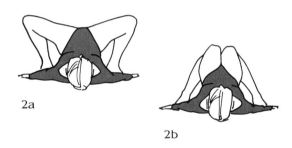

2a

2b

1. Lie on your back, knees bent, feet and knees parallel and a little more than hip-distance apart. Raise your pelvis and lower slightly as you release the muscle. Do not touch the floor with your buttocks during the exercise. The movement is small but very concentrated. As you lift up, squeeze the buttocks muscles. Be careful not to let your back arch. Continue this raising and lowering in a rhythmic motion until the muscle begins to burn.

2. Place your feet wider apart. Bring the knees farther apart as you release the buttocks; press the knees together as you push the buttocks up and squeeze. Continue this opening and closing of the knees, resisting the motion as you close the knees and squeezing hard as you lift the buttocks. Keep a steady and rhythmic tempo going for as long as you can. *Be careful not to arch your back.*

SEPTEMBER

	MORNING	AFTERNOON
10 MONDAY		
11 TUESDAY		
12 WEDNESDAY		
13 THURSDAY		
14 FRIDAY		
15 SATURDAY		
16 SUNDAY		

Exercise—Buttocks
Health Challenge—Eliminate Processed Foods

GROIN AND HIP STRETCH

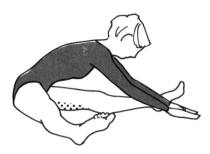

Sit with your legs spread a comfortable distance apart. Slowly lean forward from your hips, keeping your hands out in front for balance. Don't round your back or drop your head. The movement is from the hips. The back must be straight, the backs of the knees pressed into the floor. Hold and release. Remember to breathe normally. After stretching to the center, repeat to the right and to the left.

SEPTEMBER

	MORNING	AFTERNOON
17 MONDAY		
18 TUESDAY		
19 WEDNESDAY		
20 THURSDAY		
21 FRIDAY		
22 SATURDAY		
23 SUNDAY		

Exercise—Buttocks
Health Challenge—Eliminate Processed Foods

Stuffed Chard Leaves

16 *large leaves Swiss chard*
2½ *cups cooked brown rice*
 1 *onion, chopped*
 ¼ *cup oil*
1½ *cups low-fat cottage cheese*
 1 *egg, beaten*
 ½ *cup chopped parsley*
 ¾ *cup raisins*
 1 *teaspoon dill weed*

Preheat oven to 350°. Sauté onion in oil. Mix all ingredients except chard.

Wash and dry chard leaves and remove stems. Place 2 tablespoons of filling on the underside of the leaf, a third of the way from the bottom. Fold over the sides of the leaf and roll up into a square packet. Place seam-side down in a greased casserole. Cover and bake for about 30 minutes, or steam in a steamer basket over boiling water until the leaves are tender, about 20 minutes. Bake any extra filling and serve with stuffed leaves. Serves 6 to 8.

SEPTEMBER

	MORNING	AFTERNOON
24 MONDAY		
25 TUESDAY		
26 WEDNESDAY		
27 THURSDAY	ROSH HASHANAH	
28 FRIDAY		
29 SATURDAY		
30 SUNDAY		

Exercise—Buttocks
Health Challenge—Eliminate Processed Foods

Vegetable-Soybean Loaf

1 *cup raw carrots, grated*
1 *cup soybeans, cooked*
1 *cup raw beets, grated*
1 *onion, grated*
1 *green pepper, minced*
3 *tablespoons soy flour*
½ *cup wheat germ (about)*
⅓ *cup tomato juice (about)*
2 *eggs*
3 *tablespoons nutritional yeast (optional)*
1 *teaspoon oregano*

Blend all ingredients. If too dry, add more to-mato juice; if too moist, more wheat germ. Turn into oiled loaf pan. Bake at 350° for about 1 hour. Serves 6.

OCTOBER

S	M	T	W	T	F	S
	1	2	3	4	5	6
7	8	9	10	11	12	13
14	15	16	17	18	19	20
21	22	23	24	25	26	27
28	29	30	31			

EXERCISE—
THIGHS

Quad and Ankle Toner
Jazz Stretch
Quad and Knee Stretch
Thigh Stretch

HEALTH CHALLENGE—
ELIMINATE CARBONATED DRINKS

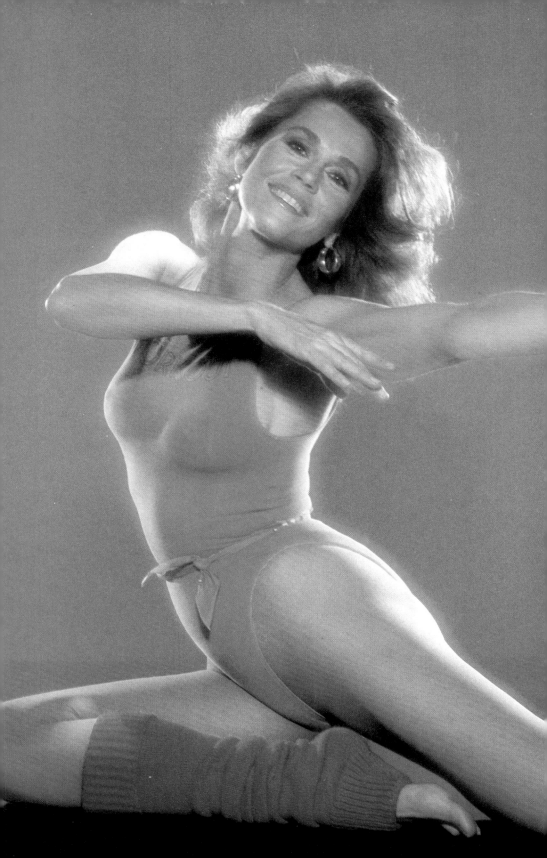

OCTOBER

Exercise—THIGHS

The quadriceps muscle in the front of the thigh runs between the kneecap and the hip. A strong thigh muscle helps protect the fragile knee joint, prevents "sagging" knees and develops good-looking muscle definition in the thigh.

Health Challenge—ELIMINATE CARBONATED DRINKS

Soda pop is a main staple of the American diet—to our detriment! Soda pop is high in sugar, often contains caffeine, artificial colorings, flavorings, and carbonation, all of which can harm our bodies. Under pressure from a more health-conscious consumer, the soda pop companies are plugging their new caffeine- and sugar-free brands, but the fact remains: they're still colored, flavored, artificially carbonated and are empty of nutrients. So why not spend this month trying out some alternatives to soda pop?

OCTOBER

	MORNING	AFTERNOON
1 MONDAY		
2 TUESDAY		
3 WEDNESDAY		
4 THURSDAY		
5 FRIDAY		
6 SATURDAY	YOM KIPPUR	
7 SUNDAY		

Exercise—Thighs
Health Challenge—Eliminate Carbonated Drinks

QUAD AND ANKLE TONER

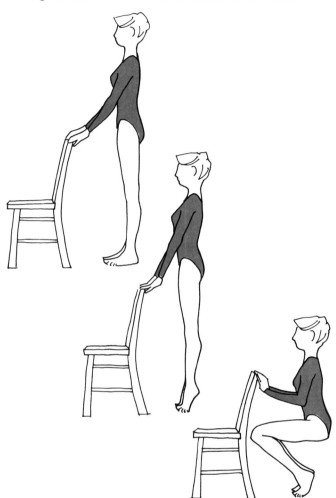

Stand facing a chair, table or wall—anything to help you balance. Place your feet parallel to each other about six inches apart. Holding lightly on to your support, rise up very high on your toes, keeping your stomach flat, buttocks tight and back straight. Then bend your knees and slowly lower your body as far as you can, staying high on your toes. Come back up, still high on your toes. Let your ankles, calves and thighs do the work. When you have straightened your legs again, lower your heels and repeat the exercise until you feel your thigh muscles begin to tire.

OCTOBER

	MORNING	AFTERNOON
8 MONDAY	COLUMBUS DAY OBSERVED	
9 TUESDAY		
10 WEDNESDAY		
11 THURSDAY		
12 FRIDAY	COLUMBUS DAY	
13 SATURDAY		
14 SUNDAY		

Exercise—Thighs
Health Challenge—Eliminate Carbonated Drinks

JAZZ STRETCH

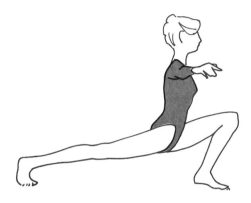

Lunge forward with the front foot flat on the floor, turned slightly out, and back leg as far behind you as possible, with the back foot facing straight ahead and toes curled forward. Arms are extended to the side, shoulder height. Gently bounce with very small bounces for 10 to 15 counts. Pause and repeat. Then repeat the exercise to the other side.

OCTOBER

	MORNING	AFTERNOON
15 MONDAY		
16 TUESDAY		
17 WEDNESDAY		
18 THURSDAY		
19 FRIDAY		
20 SATURDAY		
21 SUNDAY		

Exercise—Thighs
Health Challenge—Eliminate Carbonated Drinks

QUAD AND KNEE STRETCH

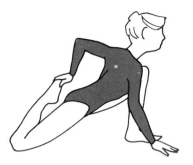

Squat down with the left foot forward flat on the floor and the right leg stretched back with the knee on the floor. Reach behind with your left hand and hold your right foot, then gently pull your heel toward your buttocks. Don't reach your buttocks back to meet your heel—keep your hips forward. Hold for thirty seconds, release and repeat to the other side.

OCTOBER

	MORNING	AFTERNOON
22 MONDAY		
23 TUESDAY		
24 WEDNESDAY		
25 THURSDAY		
26 FRIDAY		
27 SATURDAY		
28 SUNDAY		

Exercise—Thighs
Health Challenge—Eliminate Carbonated Drinks

THIGH STRETCH

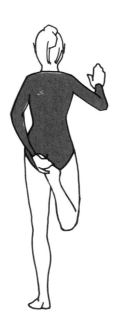

Stand and balance yourself by holding on to something with one hand. Bend your right knee and grab your foot with your left hand. Gently press your foot into your buttocks. Be careful to keep your buttocks pressing forward all the while. Repeat with opposite foot.

OCTOBER/NOVEMBER

	MORNING	AFTERNOON
29 MONDAY		
30 TUESDAY		
31 WEDNESDAY	HALLOWEEN	
1 THURSDAY		
2 FRIDAY		
3 SATURDAY		
4 SUNDAY		

Exercise—Thighs
Health Challenge—Eliminate Carbonated Drinks

Soda Substitute

Try mixing fruit concentrates (available in health food stores and some supermarkets) such as cranberry, cherry or apple concentrates with Perrier water or other natural sparkling mineral waters. Adding sparkling mineral water to any fresh fruit juice is a very pleasant refreshment.

Deer Milk

   1 *qt. water*
1½ *cups skim milk, powdered*
   3 *tablespoons corn oil*
   2 *tablespoons honey*
Dab of nutmeg, vanilla, or any other spice you like

Put all ingredients in a blender with a few ice cubes, and whip up.

NOVEMBER

S	M	T	W	T	F	S
				1	2	3
4	5	6	7	8	9	10
11	12	13	14	15	16	17
18	19	20	21	22	23	24
25	26	27	28	29	30	

EXERCISE—
ANKLES AND CALVES

Toning the Ankles and Calves
Heel Lifts
Hamstring/Achilles' Tendon Stretch

HEALTH CHALLENGE—
REDUCE CAFFEINE

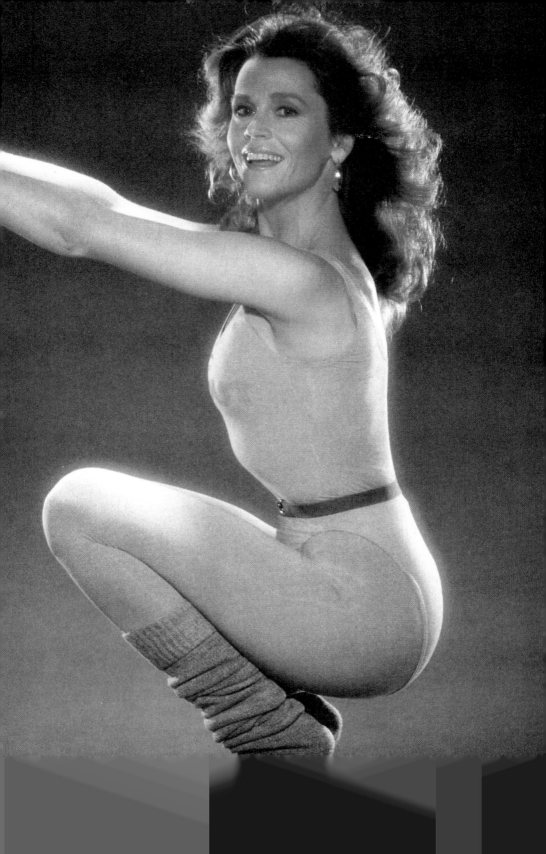

Exercise—ANKLES AND CALVES

Needless to say, the muscles in the ankles and calves get continual use and consequently are often well-defined and trim. For those who want to slim their ankles and create more definition in their calf muscles, the following exercises are very good.

Health Challenge—REDUCE CAFFEINE

Caffeine is a drug, a stimulant. It stimulates the cells of the stomach to produce more acid, the pancreas to produce more insulin, the adrenals to produce more adrenaline—and it's addictive. You need to drink more and more to feel the same effect and when you quit drinking it you can experience withdrawal symptoms—severe headaches and fatigue.

It takes quite a while for your body to stabilize itself and find energy through enough sleep, proper diet, and exercise instead of with an artificial stimulant. Ideally, you should try to stop drinking coffee altogether, as well as colas and teas that contain caffeine. Switch to delicious herbal teas. Up until now I haven't always followed my own advice and while I have greatly reduced my coffee drinking, there are still some days when I drink one, maybe two cups of the stuff. I'll join with you this month and try to cut out caffeine altogether.

OCTOBER/NOVEMBER

	MORNING	AFTERNOON
29 MONDAY		
30 TUESDAY		
31 WEDNESDAY		
1 THURSDAY		
2 FRIDAY		
3 SATURDAY	SADIE HAWKINS' DAY	
4 SUNDAY		

Exercise—Ankles and Calves
Health Challenge—Reduce Caffeine

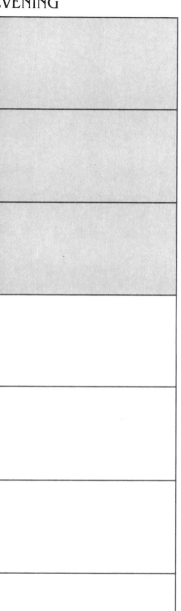

TONING THE ANKLES AND CALVES

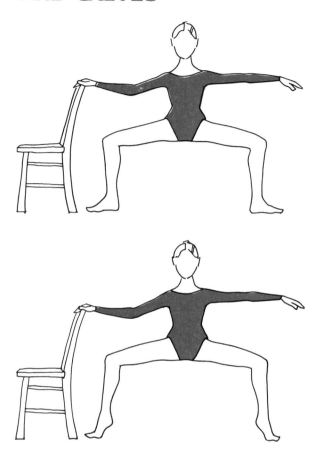

Hold on to a chair, table or railing. Stand with your legs *wide* apart, feet turned out. The wider the stance, the more benefit you'll get out of the movement. Bend your knees and lower yourself so that your buttocks are almost level with your knees. Now raise your heels as high as you can lift them, then lower them to the floor. When doing this, don't rush and don't move your hips—only your heels. Try to keep your hips on a line with your knees. Continue in a steady tempo until your thigh muscles burn. Shake your legs out and do it again. Keep trying to increase the number of repetitions.

159

NOVEMBER

	MORNING	AFTERNOON
5 MONDAY		
6 TUESDAY	ELECTION DAY	
7 WEDNESDAY		
8 THURSDAY		
9 FRIDAY		
10 SATURDAY		
11 SUNDAY	VETERANS DAY	

Exercise—Ankles and Calves
Health Challenge—Reduce Caffeine

HEEL LIFTS

Get down on your hands and knees, knees about hip-width apart, hands flat on the floor. Now, straightening your legs, walk your hands forward and lift up high on your toes, pushing your heels forward and rolling up as far as you can to the ends of your toes. Staying in this position, lower your heels to the floor, then lift them again. Repeat this up-and-down movement in a steady tempo until you feel fatigue in your calf muscles.

NOVEMBER

	MORNING	AFTERNOON
12 MONDAY		
13 TUESDAY		
14 WEDNESDAY		
15 THURSDAY		
16 FRIDAY		
17 SATURDAY		
18 SUNDAY		

Exercise—Ankles and Calves
Health Challenge—Reduce Caffeine

HAMSTRING/ACHILLES' TENDON STRETCH

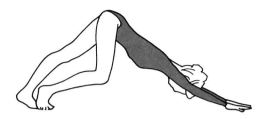

Starting on your hands and knees as in the preceding exercise but this time with your feet together, walk your hands forward. Press your left heel into the floor; release it as you press the right heel into the floor. Continue "walking" this way until you feel you've gotten a good stretch in your hamstrings.

NOVEMBER

	MORNING	AFTERNOON
19 MONDAY		
20 TUESDAY		
21 WEDNESDAY		
22 THURSDAY	THANKSGIVING DAY	
23 FRIDAY		
24 SATURDAY		
25 SUNDAY		

Exercise—Ankles and Calves
Health Challenge—Reduce Caffeine

Zucchini Oat-Flake Loaf

2 cups uncooked rolled oats
3 cups grated zucchini
½ cup grated Swiss or Cheddar cheese
2 eggs, beaten
½ cup soy meal or ½ cup wheat germ
½ cup chopped onion
3 tablespoons oil
½ cup toasted sunflower seeds
¼ teaspoon nutmeg

Preheat oven to 375°. Sauté onion in oil until soft. Combine with other ingredients and press into a well-greased loaf pan. Bake for 30 minutes. Serves 6.

No-Knead Oatmeal-Wheat Bread

2 cakes or 2 tablespoons dried yeast
3⅔ cups milk, scalded, cooled to lukewarm
½ cup honey
¼ cup oil
¼ cup raisins, seedless
¼ cup soybeans, roasted, ground
½ cup nutritional yeast (optional)
½ teaspoon mace, ground
½ cup milk powder
5 cups whole wheat flour
2 cups oatmeal

Soften cake or dried yeast in ⅔ cup milk combined with honey. Stir. Let rise and bubble for 10 minutes. Add rest of milk to oil. Blend in raisins, nutritional yeast, mace, milk powder. Add softened yeast mixture, then flour and oats, and blend thoroughly. Dough should be soft to touch but not too wet. Set bowl of dough in pan of warm water (85°F). Cover with heavy towel. Let rise in warm place for 1½ to 2 hours. Punch down. Turn into 2 oiled bread pans. Cover with towel, set in warm place and let rise about 45 minutes more. Place bread pans in cold oven, turn on heat and bake for 15 minutes, letting temperature rise to 375°; lower to 325° and bake for an additional 40 minutes. Makes 2 loaves.

NOVEMBER/DECEMBER

	MORNING	AFTERNOON
26 MONDAY		
27 TUESDAY		
28 WEDNESDAY		
29 THURSDAY		
30 FRIDAY		
1 SATURDAY		
2 SUNDAY		

Exercise—Ankles and Calves
Health Challenge—Reduce Caffeine

Tomato Soup

3 cups fresh or canned tomatoes
1 medium onion
2 stalks celery
2 tablespoons oil or margarine
1 carrot
¾ teaspoon oregano
1½ teaspoons basil
1 quart hot vegetable stock
Pepper to taste

Chop the tomatoes into small pieces if you don't mind using the skins, or simply rub them over a grater to get the juice and pulp. Chop the onion and celery and grate the carrot. Sauté the onion along with the celery and carrot until the onion is soft. Add oregano, basil and tomatoes to the pot and simmer gently for 15 minutes. If you want a smooth creamy texture, purée the soup in a blender or food mill. Add the hot stock and bring to a boil. Simmer on low heat for 5 minutes. Season with pepper. Makes 8 cups.

DECEMBER

S	M	T	W	T	F	S
						1
2	3	4	5	6	7	8
9	10	11	12	13	14	15
16	17	18	19	20	21	22
23	24	25	26	27	28	29
30	31					

EXERCISE—
WHAT YOU CAN DO AT YOUR DESK

Stretch for Lower and Upper Back
Arm and Side Stretch
Stretch for Shoulder Tension
Stretch to Relieve Pressure on Lower Back
Neck Stretch
Upper Back and Neck Stretch
Stretch for Tension in Shoulders and Upper Back

HEALTH CHALLENGE—
INCREASE YOUR INTAKE OF COMPLEX CARBOHYDRATES

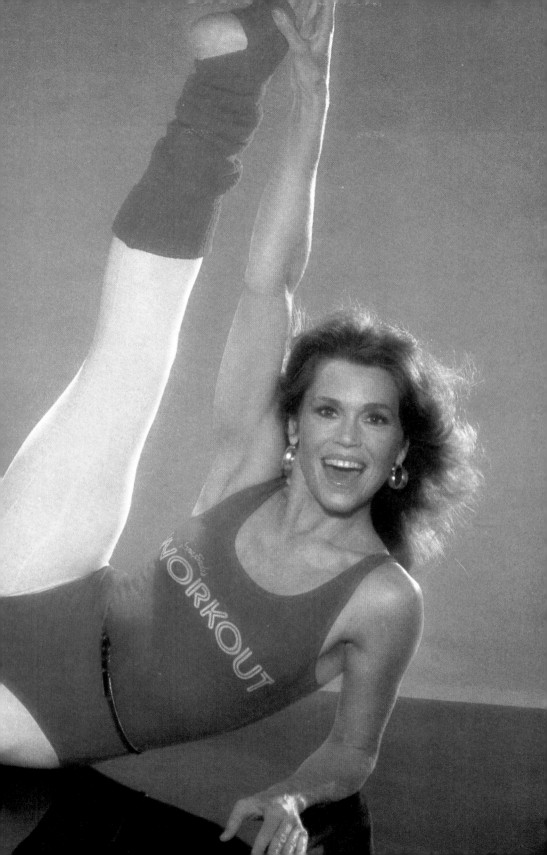

DECEMBER

Exercise—WHAT YOU CAN DO
AT YOUR DESK

Many women spend long hours at desks and work stations that are poorly designed, doing work that is stressful. Secretaries rank second highest as victims of stress-related diseases, including heart disease.

Here are some exercises you can do at your desk that will improve circulation and relieve stress and fatigue. Remember, however, your taking personal responsibility for reducing your own work-related, health-damaging stress does not shift responsibility for creating a more healthful work environment away from the companies themselves.

Health Challenge—INCREASE YOUR INTAKE OF COMPLEX CARBOHYDRATES

Snack and processed foods have created a number of significant changes in our diets, not the least of which is a decrease in the amount of complex carbohydrates we consume. This has had a major impact on our health. Complex carbohydrates, which are found in whole grains, beans, seeds and fresh vegetables, are primary sources of essential vitamins and minerals.

Complex carbohydrates are "energy" foods. They are high in fiber and are digested slowly so that their glucose enters the system gradually, giving us a steady, long-term supply of energy.

Obviously, if you are trying to lose weight you should limit the amount of bread and beans you eat, but please don't eliminate them altogether. Fiber is important for those of you who want to lose weight because it decreases the amount of calories you absorb from your food.

During these cold winter days, try starting the day with cooked cereal and not the "instant" kind that has been stripped of many nutrients. The healthy variety takes a little longer to cook but is tasty, crunchy and eminently more satisfying.

NOVEMBER/DECEMBER

	MORNING	AFTERNOON
26 MONDAY		
27 TUESDAY		
28 WEDNESDAY		
29 THURSDAY		
30 FRIDAY		
1 SATURDAY		
2 SUNDAY		

Exercise—What You Can Do at Your Desk
Health Challenge—Increase Your Intake of
Complex Carbohydrates

STRETCH FOR LOWER AND UPPER BACK

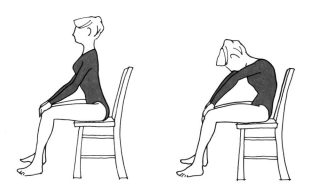

Sit on a firm chair and place your feet flat on the floor hip-distance apart. Press your lower back forward and upward, trying to lengthen the spine and lift the chest to the ceiling. Exhale as you press. Inhale and release by relaxing and slightly rounding your back and pulling your stomach inward. Do 5 times.

ARM AND SIDE STRETCH

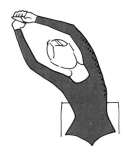

Sit up straight on a firm chair, reach arms over your head, grab your left hand with your right hand and pull your left arm over to the right side, keeping the arms from bending as much as possible. Think of pulling up out of the torso as your arms stretch to the right. Hold. Breathe. Repeat to the other side.

DECEMBER

	MORNING	AFTERNOON
3 MONDAY		
4 TUESDAY		
5 WEDNESDAY		
6 THURSDAY		
7 FRIDAY		
8 SATURDAY		
9 SUNDAY		

Exercise—What You Can Do at Your Desk
Health Challenge—Increase Your Intake of
   Complex Carbohydrates

STRETCH FOR SHOULDER TENSION

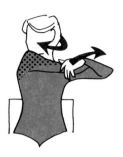

Sit up straight on a firm chair, consciously pulling up out of your torso. Place your right hand on your left shoulder. Grab your right arm above the elbow with your left hand and pull your right elbow as far over to the left as you can while looking over your right shoulder. Hold for a good stretch. Breathe. Release. Repeat to the other side.

STRETCH TO RELIEVE PRESSURE ON LOWER BACK

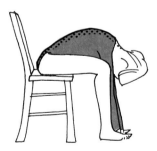

Sit in a firm chair, feet flat on the floor. Drop forward over your knees; let your arms hang down. Hold for fifty seconds and breathe deeply. Roll back up, one vertebra at a time, and repeat.

DECEMBER

	MORNING	AFTERNOON
10 MONDAY		
11 TUESDAY		
12 WEDNESDAY		
13 THURSDAY		
14 FRIDAY		
15 SATURDAY		
16 SUNDAY		

Exercise—What You Can Do at Your Desk
Health Challenge—Increase Your Intake of
   Complex Carbohydrates

NECK STRETCH

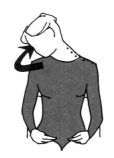
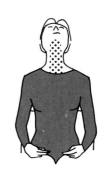
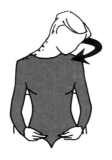
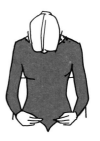

Sit up straight but relaxed, pulling up out of the torso, shoulders relaxed, stomach pulled in. Slowly roll your head in a full circle to the left 2 times and then to the right 2 times. Feel a good stretch in the neck. Don't rush and don't let the shoulders hunch up. Don't forget to breathe.

DECEMBER

	MORNING	AFTERNOON
17 MONDAY		
18 TUESDAY		
19 WEDNESDAY	HANUKKAH, FIRST DAY	
20 THURSDAY		
21 FRIDAY		
22 SATURDAY		
23 SUNDAY		

Exercise—What You Can Do at Your Desk
Health Challenge—Increase Your Intake of
   Complex Carbohydrates

UPPER BACK AND NECK STRETCH

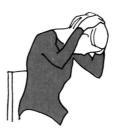

Sit up straight on a chair. Place your fingers behind your head and gently press your chin down to your chest, allowing your elbows to come forward alongside your head. Keep pressing, breathing steadily. Release. Try to hold this position for a minute or two and see if you don't feel more awake and alert when you're through.

STRETCH FOR TENSION IN SHOULDERS AND UPPER BACK

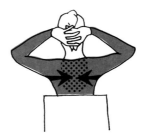

Sitting up straight as before, place your hands behind your head with fingers laced, elbows out to the side. With your head up, squeeze your shoulder blades tightly together. Hold, breathing steadily. Release. Repeat several times.

DECEMBER

	MORNING	AFTERNOON
24 MONDAY		
25 TUESDAY	CHRISTMAS DAY	
26 WEDNESDAY		
27 THURSDAY		
28 FRIDAY		
29 SATURDAY		
30 SUNDAY 31 MONDAY		

Exercise—What You Can Do at Your Desk
Health Challenge—Increase Your Intake of
 Complex Carbohydrates

Rye and Lentil Pilaf

½ cup rye
½ cup lentils
1 small onion, minced
½ cup diced carrot
½ cup diced celery
1 tablespoon oil
1 teaspoon caraway seeds (optional)
¼ teaspoon thyme
¼ teaspoon sage
3 cups chicken stock
Pepper to taste

Cook rye and lentils according to preferred method. Drain. (Liquid may be reserved for a soup base.) Sauté onion, carrot and celery in oil until tender. Combine with cooked rye and lentils, add herbs and chicken stock. Season to taste, cover and steam for 10 minutes or until hot. Serves 4.

All-in-One Cereal

2 cups cracked wheat
1 cup rolled oats
½ cup toasted wheat germ
½ cup raw wheat germ
½ cup soy grits
½ cup wheat bran
1 cup coarse cornmeal

Mix all ingredients together. Bring 4 cups water to a boil and pour 1 cup of the combined cereal in slowly. Cook and stir for a minute or two, then cover and cook over *very* low heat (a double boiler is ideal) for 20 to 25 minutes. Milk may be used in place of water. Makes 4 cups cooked cereal.

Store the balance of the uncooked mixture in a cool place to use another day.

EXERCISE REFERENCE CHART

ARMS

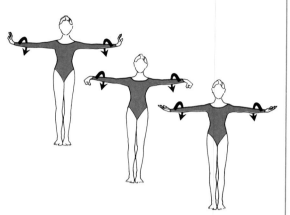

ARM CIRCLES

Stand with feet together, arms stretched out to the side just below shoulder level and slightly forward. Shoulders should be relaxed, stomach pulled in, buttocks squeezed tight. Circle both arms to the back 24 times with your hands flexed upward, 24 times with your knuckles flexed downward, 24 times with palms cupped upward.

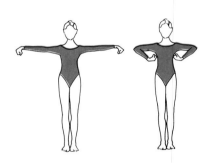

DELTOID SWING

Stand with feet together, arms stretched out to the side, shoulder height, fists dropped down. In a steady, rhythmic tempo, bend your elbows bringing the fists in toward your body, breast height, and then out again. Keep your upper arms shoulder height the entire time.

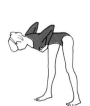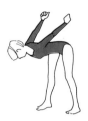

TRICEPS LIFTS

Stand with feet wide apart (you may bend your knees slightly). Bend forward, keeping your back flat, until your torso is parallel to the floor. Make fists with both hands close to your shoulders, elbows bent alongside your torso and pointing upward. Then straighten your arms and stretch them as high as possible behind you without letting them go out to the sides. Bring them in again and repeat this movement at a fairly rapid and rhythmic tempo until your muscles tire.

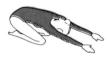

PRAYING MANTIS

Sit back on your heels, knees hip-distance apart. Bend forward, placing your forehead and hands, palms down, on the floor. Slide or walk your forearms as far forward as you can while keeping your back and neck in a straight line. You should be looking toward your feet. You can increase the stretch by reaching forward alternately with one arm then the other, but keep your hips down on your heels and your forehead on the floor. Hold at the extreme position of the stretch then release.

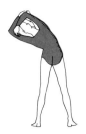

TRICEPS AND SHOULDER STRETCH

Stand with your feet a little more than hip-distance apart. Bring your arms up, crossing them behind your head and grasping each elbow with your hands. Gently pull your right elbow with the left hand as you bend slowly to the left side from your hips. You may bend your knees slightly. *Be sure your hips are forward and that your torso bends directly to the side without leaning forward—and don't arch your back.* Repeat to opposite side.

PECTORALS

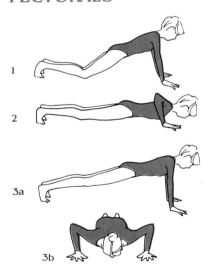

PUSH-UPS

1. Start on your hands and knees with toes on the floor, hands parallel to each other a little more than shoulder-width apart. The wider apart your hands are, the more you work your pectoral muscles.

2. Keeping your knees on the floor, lower your body straight down as far as you can, then push yourself straight up to the starting position. Continue until your muscles tire. *Concentrate on keeping your back flat.*

Don't let your buttocks stick up. Inhale as you lower, exhale as you push up.

3. As you develop strength in your arms and chest, try straight-leg push-ups.

Start slowly. Increase the number of push-ups gradually.

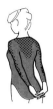
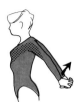

SHOULDER AND CHEST STRETCH

Stand with feet a few inches apart. Clasp your hands behind your back and, keeping your arms straight, lift them up behind you until you feel a stretch in the shoulders and chest. Hold, keeping your chest out, chin in and shoulders down.

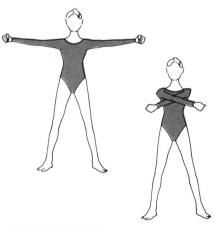

FRONT ARM CROSS

Stand up very straight with feet wide apart, stomach pulled in, buttocks tight and arms out to sides. Starting at waist height, criss-cross (cross, then open) your straight arms in front of your body with closed fists facing inward. Continue criss-crossing straight arms while raising them above your head, then lowering them slowly back down to waist level. Repeat 6 times. Then do 20 criss-crosses with arms at shoulder-height. The wider you open your arms before crossing them, the more you work your pectorals.

WAIST

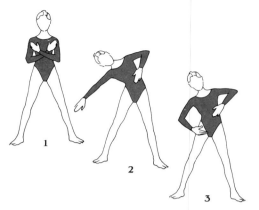

1

2

3

SIDE PULLS

1. Stand with your feet a little more than hip-distance apart, stomach pulled in, buttocks tight, hands crossed in front of your torso, palms facing your body.

2. Pull over to the right, reaching down and out with your right arm while your left elbow bends upward as far as it can go. You should feel a pull up the left side of your body. Let your head relax to the right. Keep your left shoulder back and your hips forward.

3. Come back up almost into the starting position. This down-and-up movement is done to one count. Do 10 to 20 counts to the right and then repeat to the left.

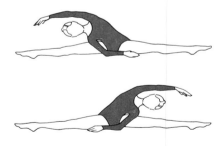

OPEN STRIDE FLOOR STRETCH

Sit on the floor with your legs as far apart as you can without feeling strained, keeping the backs of your knees pressed into the floor. Toes pointed. Lengthen your torso out of your hips and then reach to the right with the left arm overhead, keeping both hips on the floor and legs turned out. Reach as far to the right as you can, arm over the ear. Hold the stretch, breathe, return to the center and repeat to the other side. Continue the exercise until you have felt a good stretch.

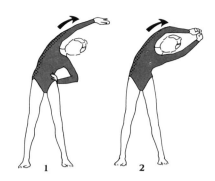

1

2

STANDING WAIST STRETCH

1. Stand with your feet a little more than hip-distance apart. With your left hand on your hip, reach your right hand over your head and slowly bend at your waist to the left side. Hold, breathe, feel a good stretch. Return to center and repeat to the other side.

2. The next time you stretch to the side, instead of putting your hand on your hip, grab your right hand with your left hand and then bend slowly to the left, keeping your hips forward and your shoulders facing front. Hold the stretch, breathe, relax, return to center and repeat to the other side. Try to increase the time you hold each stretch. *Do not bounce.* Repeat until you feel well stretched.

ABDOMINALS

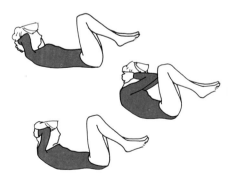

ABDOMINAL CURL

Lie on your back with knees bent and lifted toward your chest. Clasp your hands behind your head and, keeping your chin tucked in and elbows forward alongside your ears, lift your head and shoulders until your elbows touch your knees. Release slightly (don't let your head and shoulders touch the floor) and lift again. Exhale as you lift, inhale as you release. Repeat as many times as you can in a steady, rhythmic tempo.

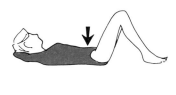

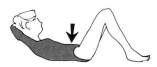

BENT-KNEE SIT-UPS

Lie down with your knees bent, feet a little more than hip-distance apart, toes and knees parallel, hands clasped behind your head with elbows back, chin up. Contract your stomach muscles by pushing the lower back into the floor, then lift your upper body several inches. Hold a second and release slightly but don't lower all the way to the floor; then lift again. Exhale as you lift, inhale as you release. Do as many times as you can in a steady, rhythmic tempo.

There are several things to bear in mind when doing these Bent-Knee Sit-ups:

1. Your head and neck should be relaxed. Don't hold your head up with the neck but let your hands and arms support it.
2. Don't tuck your chin in; look up at the ceiling, not at your knees.
3. Keep your elbows back.
4. Don't use your arms to lift your upper body. You lift by contracting inward. Think of pushing a penny into the floor with your lower back. Another image that might help is to think of someone punching you in the stomach, causing you to contract inward while your upper body lifts.

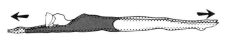

ABDOMINAL STRETCH

Lie on your back with your legs out straight and your arms extended on the floor over your head. Stretch the right arm and right leg out from the body in opposite directions, feeling a stretch up the right side. Hold for eight seconds, release and then repeat to the left. Don't let the lower back arch.

BACK

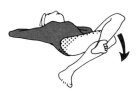

LOWER BACK AND HIP STRETCH

Lie down, place your feet flat on the floor and your hands behind your head, elbows resting on the floor. Cross your left leg over your right leg. Let the weight of your left leg press your right leg as far over to the left as you can, keeping your elbows, shoulders and upper back flat on the floor. Stretch, breathe, and don't tense. Hold for forty seconds, then release. Repeat to the other side, with the right leg crossed over the left leg and pressing down to the right.

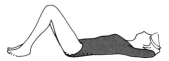

LOWER BACK STRETCH

Lying on your back with knees bent, feet flat on the floor a little more than hip-distance apart and hands behind your head, squeeze your buttocks as you push your lower back into the floor and tighten your abdominal muscles. Hold this contraction ten seconds, release and repeat again a number of times.

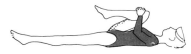

BACK STRETCH

Lie flat on your back with legs straight. Bend your right knee, grasp with both hands and gently pull it toward your chest, keeping the back of your neck pressed into the floor. Hold for forty seconds. Lower the leg and repeat with the left one.

SQUAT

Squat with your feet flat and slightly turned out, heels about one foot apart. Arms should be inside the knees, putting gentle pressure on the knees to keep them from rolling in. Knees should be directly above the toes. Hold for as long as is comfortable.

HIPS AND UPPER THIGHS

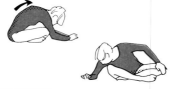

HIP STRETCH

Sit up straight with your legs crossed, right leg in front of your left. Now round your back down over your legs until you feel a good stretch in your back and hips. Try to place your elbows on the floor in front of you. Now round your back down over the right knee until you feel a good stretch, breathe, hold, release and sit up. Recross your legs so the left leg is in front. Repeat, rounding down in front then to the side over your left knee.

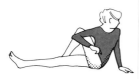

LOWER BACK AND HIP STRETCH

Sit with your right leg straight ahead and flat on the floor. Bend your left leg, cross your left foot over and place it down flat outside your right knee. Bend your right elbow and rest it on the outside of your upper left thigh just below the knee. Place your left hand behind you and slowly turn your head and upper body to look over your left shoulder. As you do this, gently press your right elbow in the opposite direction against your left thigh. Hold, breathe easily, repeat to the other side.

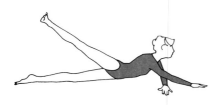

BACK OF HIPS

Lie on your stomach, raise your head and chest off the floor and support yourself on your elbows. Lift your right leg as high as you can, then lower it several inches, but without touching the floor. This is a small movement, lifting from a lifted position. Concentrate on working the back of the hip. Continue this lift until your hip muscle tires.

Then repeat with the left leg. This exercise also strengthens muscles of the back. If you have any history of back problems or are over fifty, do this exercise with your chest on the floor.

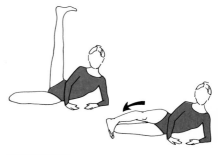

CROSSOVERS

Lie on your left side with your head and torso raised and supported by your left elbow. Flex the left knee so that the thigh is in a line with your torso and raise the right leg straight up with the foot flexed. Keeping your hips still and your knees straight, lower your leg in front of you at a comfortable angle to about three inches above the floor, then lift it up again. Continue this movement with a steady rhythm until the hip muscle tires. Then repeat to the other side. It is important when lifting the leg not to let your hips rock backward to help you. Imagine there is a wall behind your hips pressing them forward and a friend is pulling your right foot away from your body as you lower your leg. It is stretched so far out from your body that you need your right hand on the floor in front of you for balance. Inhale as you lower your leg, exhale as you raise it.

INNER THIGHS

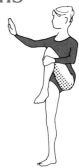

STANDING STRETCH

Stand on one leg with your hand resting on something for support. Grasp your knee with the other hand and pull it to your chest while keeping your back straight and your hips under. Bend your standing leg slightly and point your toes straight ahead. Hold, then repeat to the other side.

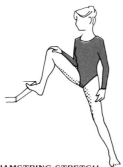

GROIN AND HAMSTRING STRETCH

Stand and place the toes of one foot on something solid about table height with your heel stretching down. Hold on to something for balance, if necessary. Turn the foot of the standing leg out, parallel to the support. Then bend your raised knee as you press your hips forward as far as you can without tensing. Hold, release. Repeat and then do the same thing to the other side.

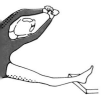

STANDING LEG AND HIP STRETCH

Place your left leg on something solid about table height. Turn the foot of the right leg so that it is parallel to the support and turn your body to face that same direction. Grasp your right wrist with your left hand and as though you were pulling your right hand and arm up and over your head, slowly bend sideways toward the raised leg, keep your upper body facing straight ahead. Hold the stretch and release slowly. Repeat with opposite leg.

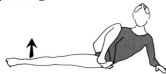

INNER THIGH LIFT

Lie on your left side, supported on your left elbow, your body in a straight line with your left leg. Cross your right leg over the left and place your toes on the floor and your right hand on the right foot. Be very sure the bottom leg is turned out with the inner thigh facing the ceiling. When you look down at your leg, you should see your inner thigh, not the top of your leg. Your weight should be directly on the left hip. Keeping your toes

pointed, lift the left leg up several inches above the floor and then lower it again without touching the floor. Repeat 10 to 20 times. Pause, flex your left foot, move it backward three inches and lift-lower again 10 to 20 times. Repeat to the other side.

BUTTOCKS

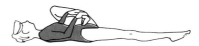

BUTTOCKS STRETCH

Lying on your back with legs straight, flex your left knee, grab your left foot with both hands, and stretch it across your groin until you feel a good stretch in the left hip. Repeat to the other side.

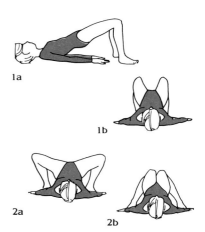

1a

1b

2a

2b

BUTTOCKS LIFT

1. Lie on your back, knees bent, feet and knees parallel and a little more than hip-distance apart. Raise your pelvis and lower slightly as you release the muscle. Do not touch the floor with your buttocks during the exercise. The movement is small but very concentrated. As you lift up, squeeze the buttocks muscles. Be careful not to let your back arch. Continue this raising and lowering in a rhythmic motion until the muscle begins to burn.

2. Place your feet wider apart. Bring the knees farther apart as you release the buttocks; press the knees together as you push the buttocks up and squeeze. Continue this opening and closing of the knees, resisting the motion as you close the knees and squeezing hard as you lift the buttocks. Keep a steady and rhythmic tempo going for as long as you can. *Be careful not to arch your back.*

BUTTOCKS *(continued)*

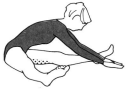

GROIN AND HIP STRETCH

Sit with your legs spread a comfortable distance apart. Slowly lean forward from your hips, keeping your hands out in front for balance. Don't round your back or drop your head. The movement is from the hips. The back must be straight, the backs of the knees pressed into the floor. Hold and release. Remember to breathe normally. After stretching to the center, repeat to the right and to the left.

THIGHS

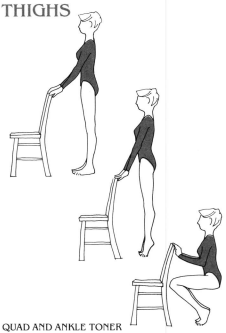

QUAD AND ANKLE TONER

Stand facing a chair, table or wall—anything to help you balance. Place your feet parallel to each other about six inches apart. Holding lightly on to your support, rise up very high on your toes, keeping your stomach flat, buttocks tight and back straight. Then bend your knees and slowly lower your body as far as you can, staying high on your toes. Come back up, still high on your toes. Let your ankles, calves and thighs do the work. When you have straightened your legs again, lower your heels and repeat the exercise until you feel your thigh muscles begin to tire.

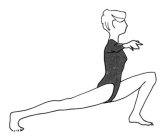

JAZZ STRETCH

Lunge forward with the front foot flat on the floor, turned slightly out, and back leg as far behind you as possible, with the back foot facing straight ahead and toes curled forward. Arms are extended to the side, shoulder height. Gently bounce with very small bounces for 10 to 15 counts. Pause and repeat. Then repeat the exercise to the other side.

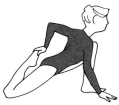

QUAD AND KNEE STRETCH

Squat down with the left foot forward flat on the floor and the right leg stretched back with the knee on the floor. Reach behind with your left hand and hold your right foot, then gently pull your heel toward your buttocks. Don't reach your buttocks back to meet your heel—keep your hips forward. Hold for thirty seconds, release and repeat to the other side.

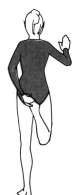

THIGH STRETCH

Stand and balance yourself by holding on to something with one hand. Bend your right knee and grab your foot with your left hand. Gently press your foot into your buttocks. Be careful to keep your buttocks pressing forward all the while. Repeat with opposite foot.

ANKLES AND CALVES

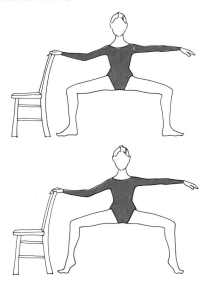

TONING THE ANKLES AND CALVES

Hold on to a chair, table or railing. Stand with your legs *wide* apart, feet turned out. The wider the stance, the more benefit you'll get out of the movement. Bend your knees and lower yourself so that your buttocks are almost level with your knees. Now raise your heels as high as you can lift them, then lower them to the floor. When doing this, don't rush and don't move your hips—only your heels. Try to keep your hips on a line with your knees. Continue in a steady tempo until your thigh muscles burn. Shake your legs out and do it again. Keep trying to increase the number of repetitions.

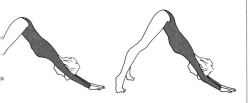

HEEL LIFTS

Get down on your hands and knees, knees about hip-width apart, hands flat on the floor. Now, straightening your legs, walk your hands forward and lift up high on your toes, pushing your heels forward and rolling up as far as you can to the ends of your toes. Staying in this position, lower your heels to the floor, then lift them again. Repeat this up-and-down movement in a steady tempo until you feel fatigue in your calf muscles.

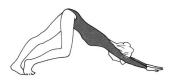

HAMSTRING/ACHILLES' TENDON STRETCH

Starting on your hands and knees as in the preceding exercise but this time with your feet together, walk your hands forward. Press your left heel into the floor; release it as you press the right heel into the floor. Continue "walking" this way until you feel you've gotten a good stretch in your hamstrings.

WHAT YOU CAN DO AT YOUR DESK

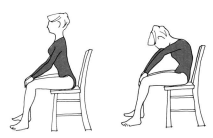

STRETCH FOR LOWER AND UPPER BACK

Sit on a firm chair and place your feet flat on the floor hip-distance apart. Press your lower back forward and upward, trying to lengthen the spine and lift the chest to the ceiling. Exhale as you press. Inhale and release by relaxing and slightly rounding your back and pulling your stomach inward. Do 5 times.

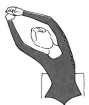

ARM AND SIDE STRETCH

Sit up straight on a firm chair, reach arms over your head, grab your left hand with your right hand and pull your left arm over to the right side, keeping the arms from bending as much as possible. Think of pulling up out of the torso as your arms stretch to the right. Hold. Breathe. Repeat to the other side.

STRETCH FOR SHOULDER TENSION

Sit up straight on a firm chair, consciously pulling up out of your torso. Place your right hand on your left shoulder. Grab your right arm above the elbow with your left hand and pull your right elbow as far over to the left as you can while looking over your right shoulder. Hold for a good stretch. Breathe. Release. Repeat to the other side.

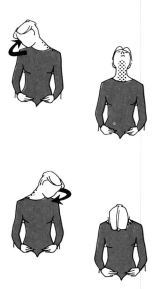

NECK STRETCH

Sit up straight but relaxed, pulling up out of the torso, shoulders relaxed, stomach pulled in. Slowly roll your head in a full circle to the left 2 times and then to the right 2 times. Feel a good stretch in the neck. Don't rush and don't let the shoulders hunch up. Don't forget to breathe.

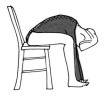

STRETCH TO RELIEVE PRESSURE ON LOWER BACK

Sit in a firm chair, feet flat on the floor. Drop forward over your knees; let your arms hang down. Hold for fifty seconds and breathe deeply. Roll back up, one vertebra at a time, and repeat.

UPPER BACK AND NECK STRETCH

Sit up straight on a chair. Place your fingers behind your head and gently press your chin down to your chest, allowing your elbows to come forward alongside your head. Keep pressing, breathing steadily. Release. Try to hold this position for a minute or two and see if you don't feel more awake and alert when you're through.

STRETCH FOR TENSION IN SHOULDERS AND UPPER BACK

Sitting up straight as before, place your hands behind your head with fingers laced, elbows out to the side. With your head up, squeeze your shoulder blades tightly together. Hold, breathing steadily. Release. Repeat several times.

The year has come to an end. Don't you feel better as a result of your new commitment to health and fitness?

Perhaps you haven't followed every health challenge to the letter. Perhaps there were times when you couldn't manage to fit exercise into your schedule. Don't be discouraged. If you managed to do half of what I've asked of you, you will have accomplished a lot.

It takes a long time to change old habits. It's hard work, and you can't expect all the results you want all at once. But please, don't stop here. Fitness is a continuing process, a journey— with steps forward and steps back—that we will make together.

In that spirit, join me in 1985 for a continuation and deepening of this progress to health.

A healthy, happy, and peaceful New Year to you from me.

1985

JANUARY
S	M	T	W	T	F	S
		1	2	3	4	5
6	7	8	9	10	11	12
13	14	15	16	17	18	19
20	21	22	23	24	25	26
27	28	29	30	31		

MAY
S	M	T	W	T	F	S
			1	2	3	4
5	6	7	8	9	10	11
12	13	14	15	16	17	18
19	20	21	22	23	24	25
26	27	28	29	30	31	

SEPTEMBER
S	M	T	W	T	F	S
1	2	3	4	5	6	7
8	9	10	11	12	13	14
15	16	17	18	19	20	21
22	23	24	25	26	27	28
29	30					

FEBRUARY
S	M	T	W	T	F	S
					1	2
3	4	5	6	7	8	9
10	11	12	13	14	15	16
17	18	19	20	21	22	23
24	25	26	27	28		

JUNE
S	M	T	W	T	F	S
						1
2	3	4	5	6	7	8
9	10	11	12	13	14	15
16	17	18	19	20	21	22
23	24	25	26	27	28	29
30						

OCTOBER
S	M	T	W	T	F	S
		1	2	3	4	5
6	7	8	9	10	11	12
13	14	15	16	17	18	19
20	21	22	23	24	25	26
27	28	29	30	31		

MARCH
S	M	T	W	T	F	S
					1	2
3	4	5	6	7	8	9
10	11	12	13	14	15	16
17	18	19	20	21	22	23
24	25	26	27	28	29	30
31						

JULY
S	M	T	W	T	F	S
	1	2	3	4	5	6
7	8	9	10	11	12	13
14	15	16	17	18	19	20
21	22	23	24	25	26	27
28	29	30	31			

NOVEMBER
S	M	T	W	T	F	S
					1	2
3	4	5	6	7	8	9
10	11	12	13	14	15	16
17	18	19	20	21	22	23
24	25	26	27	28	29	30

APRIL
S	M	T	W	T	F	S
	1	2	3	4	5	6
7	8	9	10	11	12	13
14	15	16	17	18	19	20
21	22	23	24	25	26	27
28	29	30				

AUGUST
S	M	T	W	T	F	S
				1	2	3
4	5	6	7	8	9	10
11	12	13	14	15	16	17
18	19	20	21	22	23	24
25	26	27	28	29	30	31

DECEMBER
S	M	T	W	T	F	S
1	2	3	4	5	6	7
8	9	10	11	12	13	14
15	16	17	18	19	20	21
22	23	24	25	26	27	28
29	30	31				